50 SHADES OF WHITE

VOLUME 1

Real Life Stories of Dental Implant Patients

50 SHADES OF WHITE

VOLUME 1

Real Life Stories of Dental Implant Patients

Authored by

Dr. Prem Alex Lawrence

TLC PUBLISHING INTERNATIONAL

Office Address- No. 16, 3rd Main Road, Jaganathapuram,
Velachery, Chennai 600042 (TN) India

Website: https://www.tlcpublishing.org/
Email: info.tlcpublishing@gmail.com

Published by TLC Publishing International 2024
Title : 50 SHADES OF WHITE VOLUME 1
Price : Rs.699 | $12
ISBN : 978-93-6006-375-7

First Words

In the realm of dental transformations, where smiles become narratives, and oral health is a canvas awaiting restoration, this book unfolds as a compilation of extraordinary odysseys. Each chapter encapsulates the resilience, courage, and transformative power embedded in the journeys of individuals seeking solace, confidence, and a radiant smile.

Welcome to "50 Shades of White – Volume 1". In these pages, we delve into stories that traverse continents, cultures, and the intricacies of individual lives, all converging at the pivotal intersection of dentistry and personal well-being.

Our protagonists are not just patients; they are individuals whose narratives transcend the clinical confines of dental treatment. These are tales of rediscovery, redemption, and the reclamation of confidence. As we navigate through the chapters, you'll witness the subtle artistry of dental practitioners, the resilience of patients, and the profound impact that a restored smile can have on one's life.

These stories are not just about teeth; they are about empowerment, self-assurance, and the realization that a confident smile is a gateway to a world of possibilities. As we unfold the chapters, be prepared to witness the joy, tears, and transformative power of comprehensive dental care.

I am extremely indebted to my Implant Team which includes Dr Jeyathipan, Dr Jananee, Dr Sobika, Mr Prem Valemurughan, Mrs Chithra, Dr Sathish Chandran, Dr Vijaya Nirmal, Dr Navaneetha Krishnan (Anaesthetist), Ms Nithya, Ms Bharathi, Dr Aishwarya, Ms Meenakshi, Mrs Banu, Mr Mani, Dr Rekha, Dr Renu, Mr Venu, Dr Veera who have stood by me in all my cases. Also, a huge thanks to Mr. Saravanan, my friend, who instigated me to start a YouTube channel to educate the masses about implants.

I am indebted highly to my Family - My mom, my dad, my brother, and my sister-in-law, who all stood with me during my tough times in my profession, even lending me a hand to pull me out of difficulties.

I also thank my wife and daughter for their support in creating this book, especially my daughter for naming many of my protagonists to hide their real identities.

"50 Shades of White" is a chance to discover the profound influence of dentistry on people's lives, to comprehend the delicate relationship between dentists and their patients, and to celebrate the victory of a bright, beautiful smile. Come along on this journey, where every chapter depicts strength, rejuvenation, and the happiness of a renewed smile.

Index

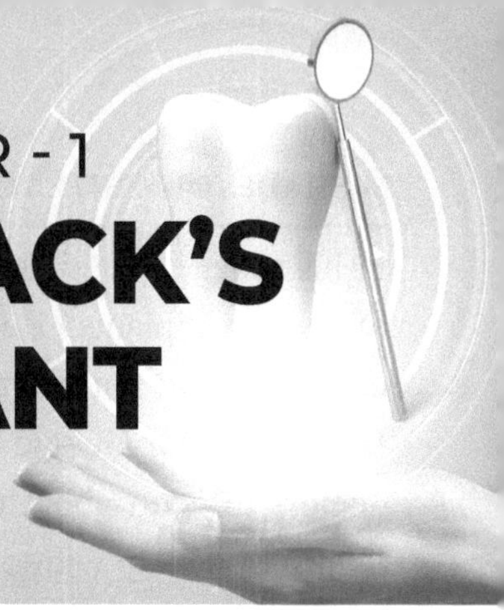

CHAPTER - 1

THE QUACK'S IMPLANT

Implants have come a long way in its design. The original design included many different shapes and sizes. There was one particular implant called TRANS MUCOSAL implant, which was unlike our traditional implant; it was adapted over the bone and not inside the bone and then restored. The usability became limited because of the cumbersome procedure, and that simpler alternative became available.

This story is of my patient from Andhra Pradesh named Mr Malli* (Name Changed), aged 34. He was a software engineer, and when he came to meet me, he had severe pain in his right lower jaw. He had no medical issues, and the only issue was that the patient had a liking for CHEAPER TREATMENTS or SERVICES.

This man lost his right lower First Molar Tooth when he was in his 20s due to decay. When he developed decay in another tooth a few years back, a dentist advised him to get this particular tooth replaced since it was an important tooth for chewing.

The story starts here. Malli went around a lot of clinics

in his village and almost did his PhD research on the cost of dental implants. He decided that implants were very costly and did not want to get a bridge. He also consulted Dr Google, Mr Google Maps, Dr Quora and many internet doctors to learn about the cost and types of implants. He finally landed up with a doctor next to his village, who was all ears. The patient recently told me that he now doubts that the doctor was an actual medical doctor.

To this doctor, Malli suggested that he could do a transmucosal implant. The doctor also thought this could be done, and they both started designing an implant. They welded a metal component to arch bars used to fix the fractured bone and very well thought this device could be used like a transmucosal implant. A truly Eureka moment.

A surgery was done with basic hardware type of screwdrivers, and this so call device was screwed onto the bone, and a crown was cemented to the device.

The actual story starts from here. The flaw in the design is one: the sterilization and technique of implantation started showing its issue in a month's time. But our Malli believed that his science project would eventually work and did not bother with the occasional pain and swelling. He used to pop in antibiotics from medical shops and managed to poke using needles whenever pus accumulated in that region.

After a few months, he thought he had gotten enough of the implant and wanted it to be removed from his mouth. But the original doctor who placed the implant refused to do so, saying it would eventually settle down, and Malli lost all confidence in himself and his scientific experiment.

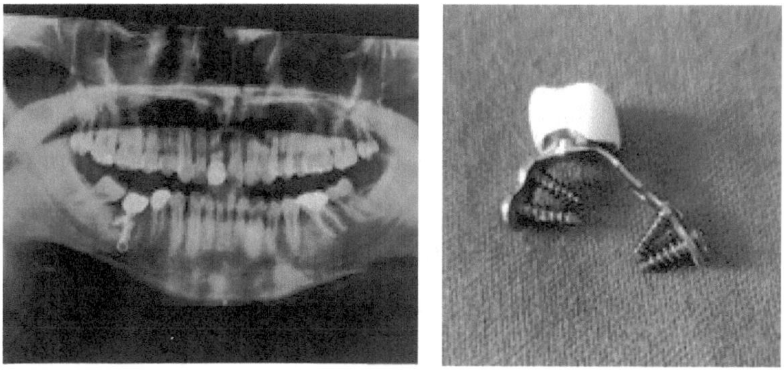

Before: The So-called Implant

He found me and landed in my clinic. Upon first assessing him, I felt he was definitely rich in Internet ideas and had now become very sceptical of dental implants or implantologists. He wanted the implant to be removed, and when I told him this was a crude implant, he was not very keen on hearing my explanation. However, eventually, we planned on removing the "IMPLANT DEVICE" and placing a regular implant on him.

The infected bone was cleaned, and it took almost an hour for me to clean and graft the region, followed by placing a regular implant near the infected site. His long turmoil was so relieved by me and my team.

He never came back for crowns when beckoned after 3 months by my team. He almost came after 2 years to get his crown in the tooth; by then, the graft I placed had taken up and good healing of our implants. And a Screw retained crown was given.

Moral of the Story:

Implantologists like me practice "Evidence-based Implantology". We practice and use devices based on prior research. People like Malli try to research the internet and word of mouth and think that they saved money by getting under-researched implants and finally end up spending more money than they intended to or undergoing huge agony over time.

Dr Google is good but does not replace or come close to any of the breathing Implantologists.

Dont be a Malli!

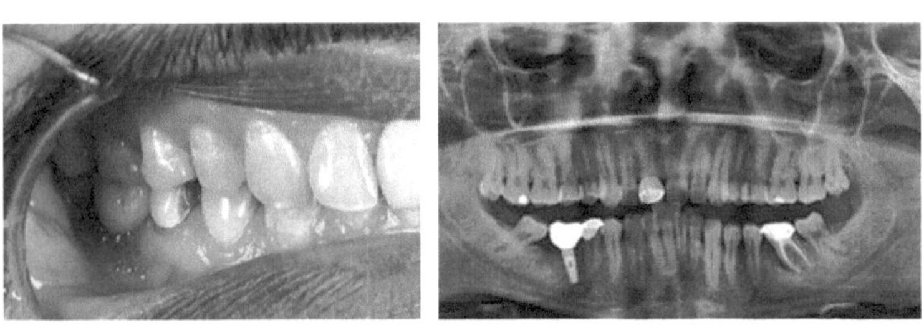

After: Corrective Implant Surgery

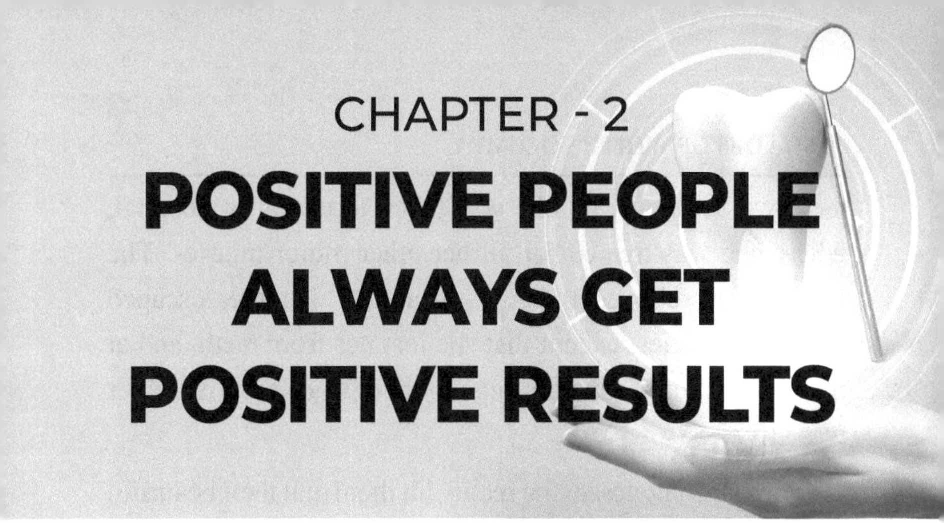

CHAPTER - 2

POSITIVE PEOPLE ALWAYS GET POSITIVE RESULTS

A smile may be infectious. I also believe Positivity can be spread across. I have an uncle, Mr Joseph Antony, who, at anything life throws at him, always remains positive, and he always looks at the positive side of life. This positivity of his has often spread to me whenever we have a chat. The next one is such a positive story.

A very beautiful girl named Aishu* (name changed), 21 years from the southern district of Tamil Nadu, landed in my clinic with a complaint of missing upper front teeth.

The story starts here. Almost a month before meeting me, Aishu was travelling on her scooter to her college one fine morning. She usually straps her helmet, and this unfortunate day, she forgot to do that or rather took it lightly. While entering a highway, her scooter was hit by a truck, and she was immediately thrown out of her vehicle.

Fortunately, or unfortunately, her helmet took the first impact; however, during the second impact, she hit her front teeth and the 3 teeth got avulsed upon impact. One of the front teeth was broken, and she was taken to a nearby hospital, where she was treated for all her other minor injuries. The family was relieved that their beautiful daughter escaped with few injuries, except that she lost her front teeth, and at that point, it didn't matter huge to them since their daughter was alive.

Once she recovered, the reality hit them that their beautiful 21-year-old daughter did not have all her upper front teeth. Imagine the trauma that the child would have undergone. She had also started going back to her college without teeth.

I still vividly remember the day I met Aishu. Though without teeth, she was always smiling. Something that spoke highly about her spirit. I knew she was a fighter. I kept complimenting her, saying that she was very positive even in this tough time. Only after all the conversations and discussions on treatment plans and when I told Aishu that she would get good, nice teeth did tears slip from her eyes, and she started crying. Though she was crying, she never left the smile. Such was the indomitable spirit of this little girl. That day, I learnt a lot about how to be positive during despair and how we will be able to overcome any hurdle with a smile.

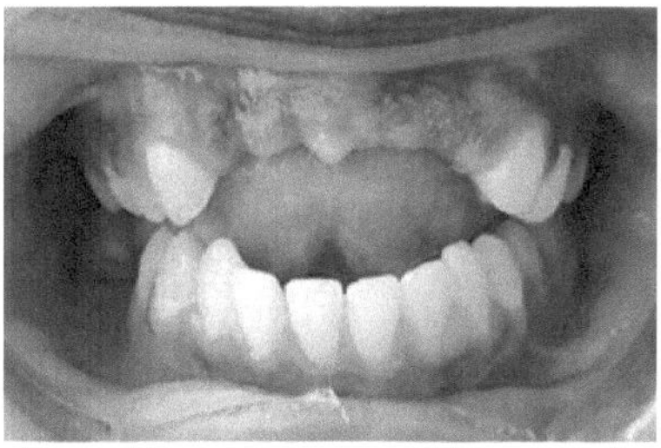

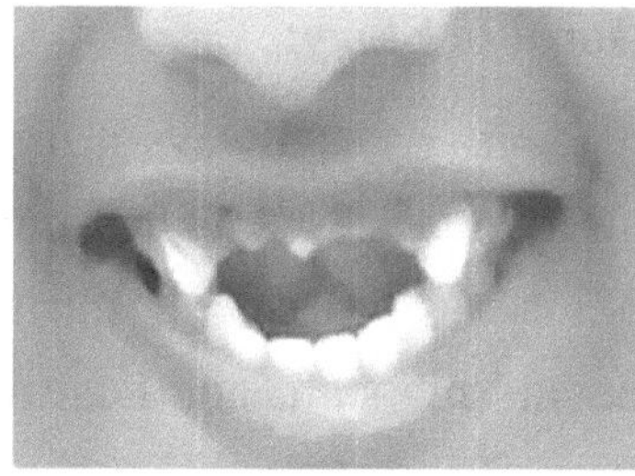

The treatment plan was tough. She had a condition called GUMMY SMILE. A Gummy smile is nothing but excessive exposure of gums when you smile, and we all now know Aishu. She smiles a lot. It was my duty to restore her smile. One more complication is that when someone loses a tooth after a trauma such as a road traffic accident, much of the bone is also lost. Hence, we will have to build back the bone as well.

I worked on bone splitting and implant placement and eventually knew I would have to replace her teeth and part of her gums as well. The surgery went well, and whatever I had planned was executed. Aishu was still smiling, always post-operatively, and the want to give my best for her also pushed me to do a perfect job.

She was on her temporaries for 4 months, and then when her Zirconia teeth came, we did multiple sittings to match her gum colour to the prosthesis, and every time, she came smiling down to the clinic. And we restored her smile to perfection.

Moral of Story:

Positivity is always infectious, and we can smile during our tough times. And learning can come from anywhere. For me, it was Aishu. Her spirit and strength were imbibed by me and my staff, and Positive people get positive things in life.

Be like Aishu! Be Positive! And always flaunt your smile! After all, we all live only once.!

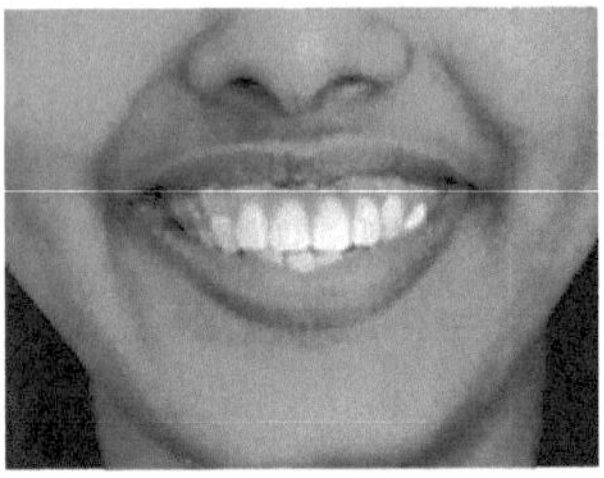
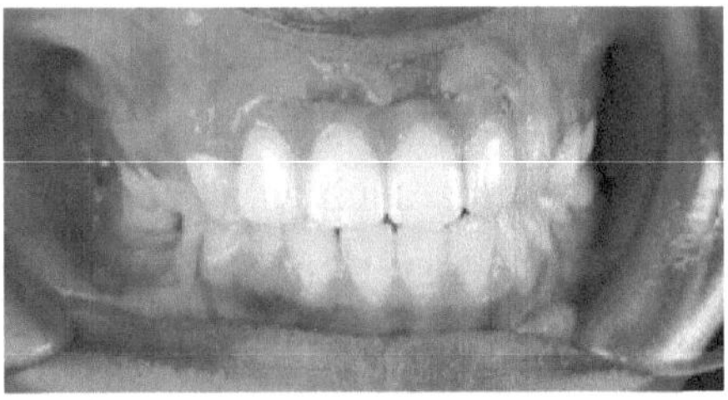

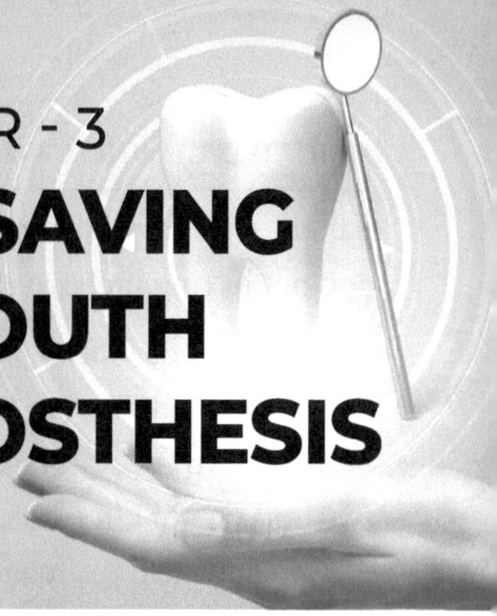

CHAPTER - 3

THE LIFE-SAVING FULL MOUTH DENTAL PROSTHESIS

The Opposite side is always Green. My Father is an extremely positive yet emotional person who is always gung-ho about life and tells me that everything happens for a reason. He also has preached to me that one bad day or one bad thing should not affect my entire life and that anything, time can heal. Such is how the next story resonates with me. In life, anything is possible, and taking one's own life is not the solution.

I still vividly remember that day when I was travelling to a car showroom to test drive a car, and on the way, I received a call from my receptionist. I was told a lady in her early 40s had called and wanted to get dental implants since all her teeth were missing, and she was wearing dentures. She also wanted to know if her problem could be sorted. She was calling from a different district, and hence, an appointment was made in the ensuing week.

That day came, and a female patient named Mrs Gayathri* (Name Changed) met me in my Clinic. She was like a typical person with no confidence, bowing her head while talking and not having any eye contact.

Gayathri has been suffering from dental issues since childhood and has undergone multiple treatments in her youth. A wrong suggestion was made to her, and for some reason, she got all her teeth removed. She thought it was not nice to have bad teeth and to wear a denture.

This is where the story turns sour and bad.

A denture is not the best treatment available for replacing a full mouth. Dentures are detrimental because they cause a lot of movement and bone loss, leading to loss of fit over the years.

But my primary issue with not retaining good teeth is for PROPRIOCEPTION. Proprioception is nothing but the ability of the teeth to perceive the quantity of forces acting on them. Tiny nerves in the ligament attached to the tooth sense even a small stone in food and avoid chewing it. This is lost when a tooth is pulled out, and any replacement cannot get this natural process back.

This is what exactly put Gayathri into depression. I was intrigued to hear the entire story. She just thought her entire problem would be solved by a denture, but the reverse happened. She was not able to eat or chew anything. The lower jaw denture was loose as well, causing embarrassment since it looked and felt bad. She also had an incident where a few of her relatives saw her without teeth.

This pushed her into depression. We started with All on Six Implants, and once the process set in, my long-time nurse, Mrs Chitra, kept conversing with her when deeper ulterior secrets came out. Gayathri has been depressed for a few months over the loss of teeth and has been contemplating ending her life a few times since she felt so helpless over this. This was a shocking revelation.

After a few months, we gave her a very good-looking full mouth with ceramic teeth over a titanium bar, and there emerged a very beautiful and confident lady. She and her family were very happy over this, and for the first time, she looked at me in the eyes to converse, and I seemingly understood how much teeth mean for someone to be confident.

This particular true story also made me feel how the work I do passionately also helps people overcome depression and even suicidal thoughts. I could understand her pain and what she was undergoing, and something that is professionally done taking a fee as well can give such satisfaction.

Moral of the Story:

Life is very precious. Nobody has the right to take their own life. Teeth may not be permanent but can be replaced. Doctors like me can help restore a beautiful smile.

Life is Precious. Period.

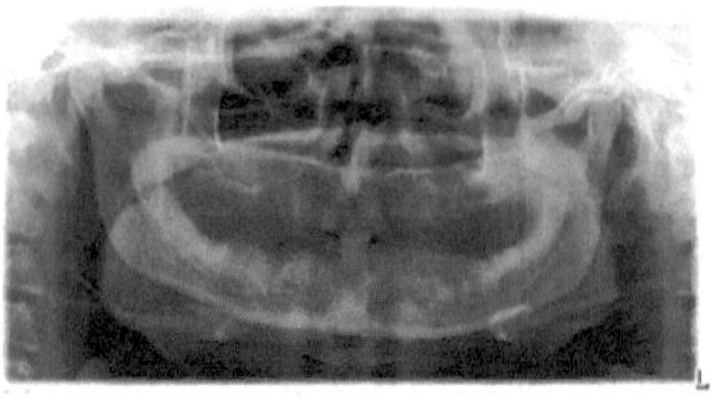

Before

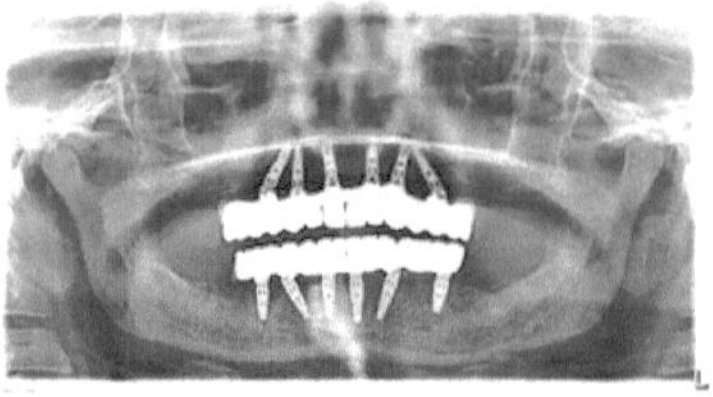

After

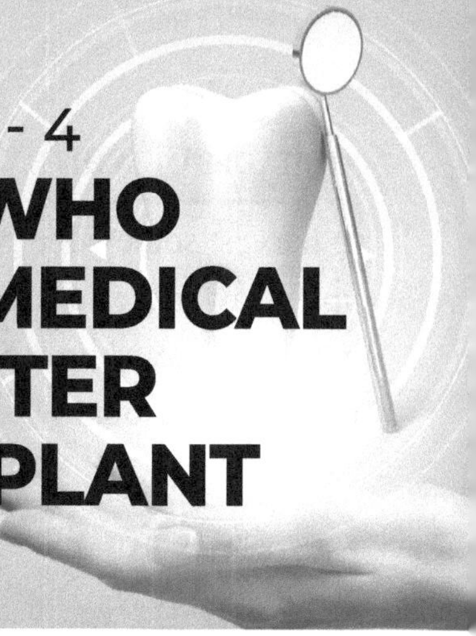

CHAPTER - 4
THE KID WHO JOINED THE MEDICAL FIELD AFTER DENTAL IMPLANT

You can instil a passion in anyone. I have had innumerable students of mine (during my stint as Assistant Professor in one Dental College) call me and inform me that they took Post Graduation in Periodontics (Gum Surgery) inspired by me. This story is about a different kind of inspiration where one of my patients wanted to be a dentist and still landed in the medical field later.

It was the summer of 2007. A young kid named Mr Ranjith* (Name Changed), barely after celebrating his 14th birthday, came up to meet me with a lost tooth. This kid's tooth shouldn't have been extracted. The dentist should have done Root canal Treatment and crown; however, Ranjith ended up getting his tooth removed. That, too, the dentist had botched up the bone so badly he came to me with a huge infected bone.

Easily, I could have advised a Bridge, but we took the tough route. We planned on reconstructing the bone using his bone from the chin. A separate surgery was performed to harvest some bone graft from his chin and attach it to the upper jaw bone to increase the quantity of bone. After six months, I gave him a beautiful zirconia crown that matched his sweet personality.

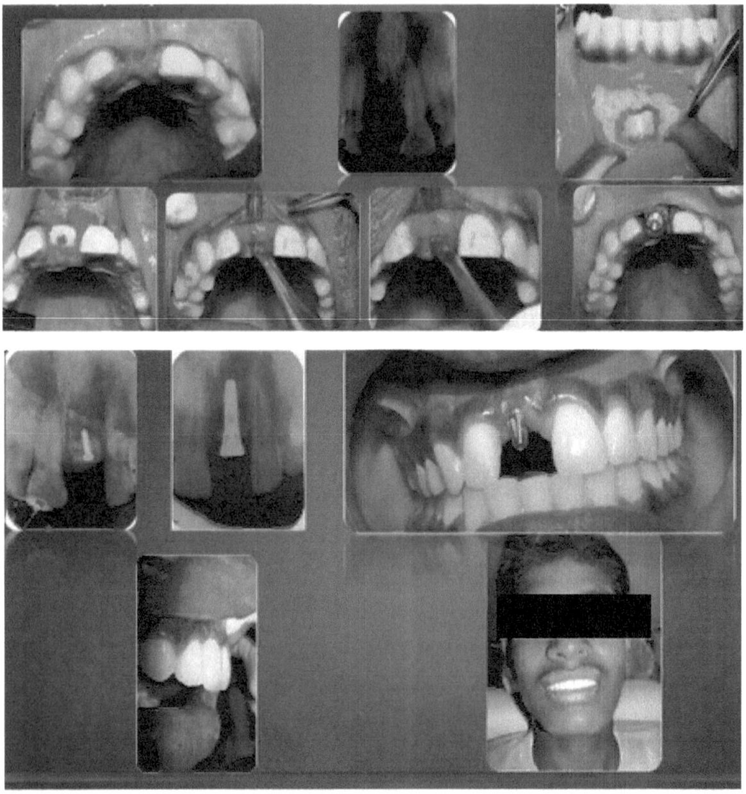

The story is during this journey of 6 months. He got so accustomed to all dental materials and staff that by the time of 6 months, he knew what procedure would be performed on him in detail. He was a regular; he knew how to place his dental bib, and at times, he even offered to hold suction from my nurse. The amount of trauma he had undergone was never a deterrent to his positive attitude. During reviews, when he wanted to join a college post-school, he and his parents came up to me and enquired whether he could take dentistry as a career.

I inquired why he wanted to be a dental surgeon, to which he answered that he had first-hand knowledge of what dentists do and, hence, he wanted to also help people like him suffering from unique issues. I was so happy that I was a source of inspiration for this kid. Eventually, he could not get through exams for dental admission, but still ended up as a male nurse.

I met him for a 12-year review a few years back, the young kid had grown into a nice man and came to invite me to his wedding, and I also came to know he was very well settled in a job in Germany. I was happy that a simple work inspired a small kid and shaped his future.

Moral of the Story:

Any medical treatment for kids always takes two opinions to avoid ending up in a soup. In this case, a botched-up extraction made the kid suffer for over a year.

Inspiration can come from anywhere! Look out!

CHAPTER - 5

THE MARRIAGE EVENT DEBACLE

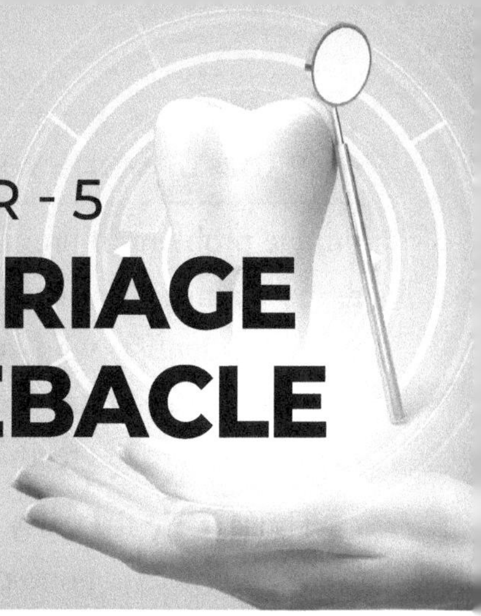

Nature is funny. Recently, I read that an Indian woman holds the Guinness record for the maximum number of teeth in the mouth, with 38 teeth. This condition is called hyperdontia (Extra Teeth). Only 3% of the world's population have such an extra tooth (minimum one). However, with evolution in work, the number of teeth is reducing due to our changes in food patterns. I have only 28 teeth, and my daughter has only 26 teeth. I proudly, at times, claim that we are ahead in Evolution (scandalous, though).

On a Funnier note, only if there was a record for no teeth present, I know many of them. The next story, though, is about a specific hyperdontia called MESIODENS. Mesiodens is nothing but an extra tooth between the upper central incisors or the Bunny teeth. This is often ugly, and the major concern is that because of its presence, the midline of the mouth is altered, or there often remains no midline.

For this story, we travel back to 2007. Mr Sekar* (Name Changed) visited me in my early days of practice with this unique problem of previously having Mesiodens. The story, as he claims, was that he wanted a correction of this and visited a dentist, who suggested he extract the Mesiodens and one of the Bunny teeth and get a flipper or a removable denture, where the teeth can be shaped accordingly.

Those were the early days of my implant practice, and I was still practising one-piece implants for anterior teeth and screw-retained crowns at a distance in Chennai at that point.

The treatment plan was simple yet complicated. This was because he was missing two teeth, but the space available was too much for one implant to be placed, and it was too little for 2 implants. It was a precarious situation since the patient was not willing to undergo orthodontic treatment to move the teeth in position since he felt he was too old, at 40 years old, to get braces.

Hence, I decided to place one implant and give two crowns. This treatment, though nowadays, I don't use it in the upper front tooth, may perform the same in the lower front teeth. But those were days, and it was a simple case and gave him nice, good ceramic teeth.

The story starts after delivering his teeth, and Sekar becomes very emotional. I was shocked to see that tears came out of a well-built 6-foot guy over a 20 mm prosthetic teeth. He asked me if he could throw his denture away. Told him to dump it in the dustbin in my room. He did it. He told me that since he had been wearing this denture for more than 10 years, he had various situations of embarrassment.

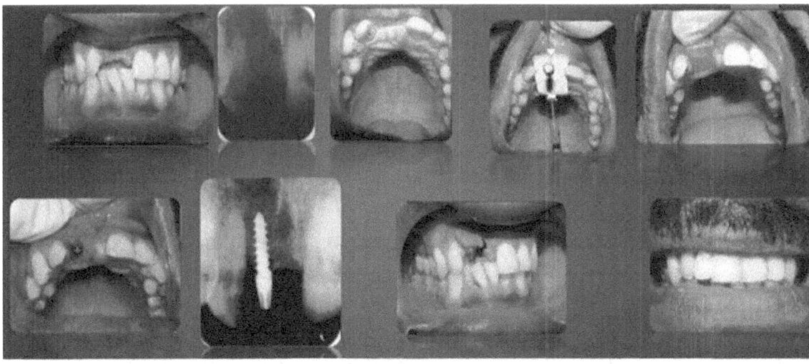

One specifically that hurt him so badly was the one at his relative's wedding, where while eating, the denture came and fell on the plantain leaf he was eating. This was seen by many of his relatives who came to know that he had false teeth and that there was one particular 5-year-old kid who insisted on seeing his artificial teeth out of his mouth since the kid thought Sekar was a magician who could take his teeth out of his mouth whereas she could not. He became a spectacle of laughter at that wedding.

He vividly remembers the hurt he underwent during that event, and that hounded him for years until now. That denture deserved nothing less than a Bin.

Moral of the Story:

Dentures are slippery and tricky. It needs to be mastered. It needs to be practised to remain in the mouth, and more practice is needed to use it for eating and chewing.

Don't be a slippery one like Sekar's Denture. Be Firm like his implants in Decisions you make in life.

Chuck Dentures! Get Fixed Teeth! Doesn't make you a Joker in front of your family and friends.

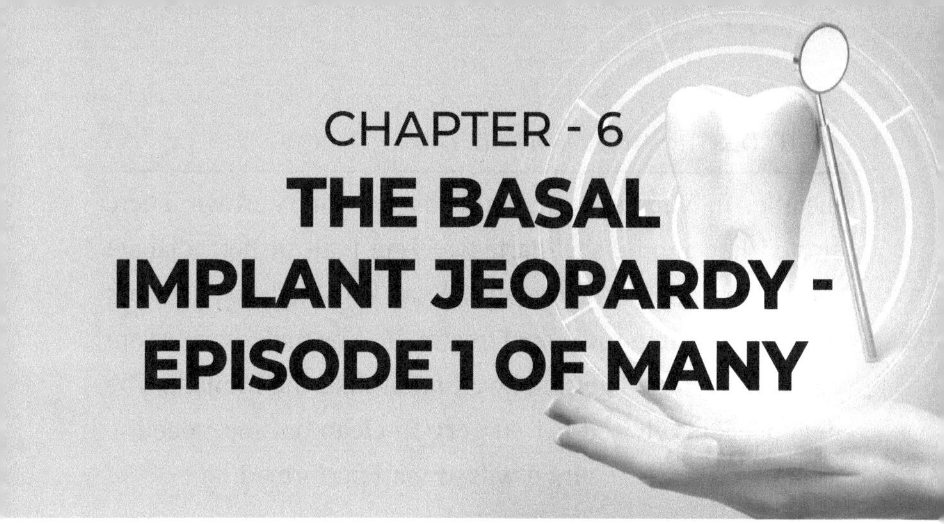

CHAPTER - 6

THE BASAL IMPLANT JEOPARDY - EPISODE 1 OF MANY

India has a huge unregulated market in terms of Implants. Such is the story with Basal Implants. Basal Implants are primitive, crude and not recognised by many regulatory bodies, including the FDA (Food and Drug Administration, USA). They are never taught in any medical school curriculum, and doctors who perform Basal implants are trained by particular companies with business interests. I have been advocating against Basal implants, having met with many patients with issues and complex problems because of basal implants.

This story is of a young girl, Ragini*(Name Changed), who came to us with her fiancee, who is also a medical lab assistant in a leading private hospital. Unfortunately, Ragini had met with an accident and lost her Right front Bunny teeth (Central Incisors). She met this doctor in Chennai who advised her to get a Basal Dental Implant and promised her that a crown could be given the same day.

Yes, the surgery was done, and a Basal implant was

installed into her jaw and sent with a temporary crown. There started her agony, she started feeling pain in her adjacent tooth. The doctor again saw her and blamed her adjacent tooth for needing root canal treatment. She underwent a root canal. She started getting swelling around the implant. The doctor again advised her surgery to clean out the infection around the implant, and it was as well performed,

Again, she developed pain in the next adjacent tooth. The doctor advised one more root canal treatment and also advised to get the adjacent two teeth out and get two more new Basal Implants. This is where her fiancee got severely fed up and then found me.

They had already spent a lakh (rupees) of money before meeting me, and I could sense their agony. I carefully examined and told them not to disturb the implant for now but to solve the problem in the adjacent tooth with a proper root canal treatment and wait and watch. This gave a solution to her pain, and never did she ever have pain. Hence, I advised her to get new crowns, and we did good crowns on the adjacent tooth as well as on the Basal Implant.

It took just 3 months for her pain in the implant to come again. This time, I wanted to examine to see if the Implant had failed and their worst dream came true, that the implant had failed along with severe mobility.

The reason is that the Basal implants do not osseointegrate or that it does not get attached to the bone. Instead, it does osseo fixation, i.e., just fixes and does not integrate. Hence, when an increased force is applied, it fails.

The toughest job was for me to clean the entire infection that had spread up to the floor of the Nose. Technically, I could not remove the entire infection since it had taken a spiral route. However, I could place a conventional endosseous implant in the site and graft the rest of the area with bone graft and wait for 4 months before giving her a fresh pair of crowns. I knew the pain they had undergone for almost a year before and made sure she and her fiance went happy, and I refrained from charging any surgeon's fee for the implant procedure.

At the time of writing this book, she is due for one more minor plastic surgery in the gums because of the gum loss due to the Basal Implant.

She got married to her fiancee now and hopes all her issues will be sorted out shortly.

Moral of the Story:

Science offers a healing touch. Do not go with unscientific methods for treating dental or, for that matter, any other ailment.

Certain treatments like Dental implants are done after years of research behind them.

Do not get Basal Implants. Ever. Period.

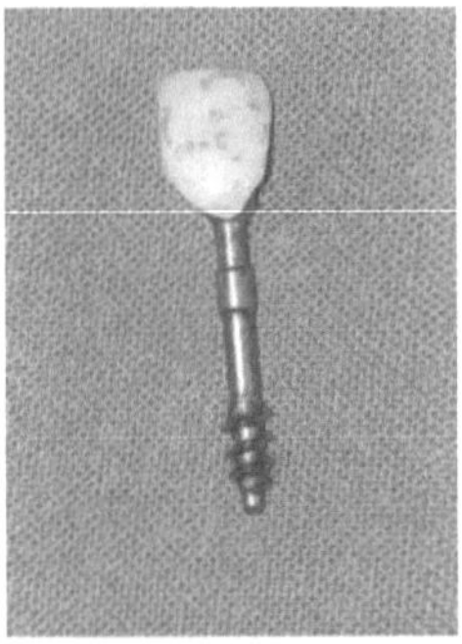

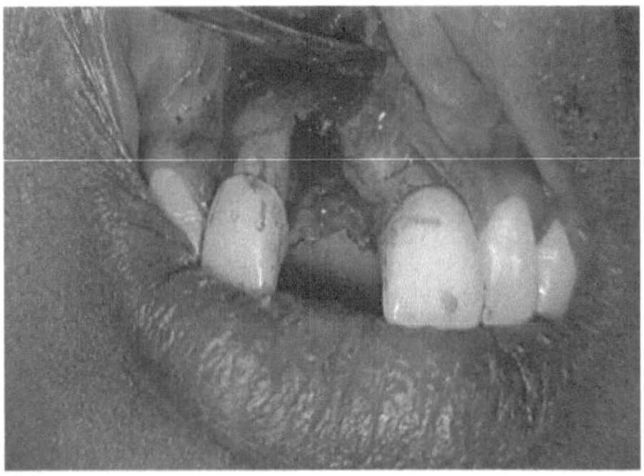

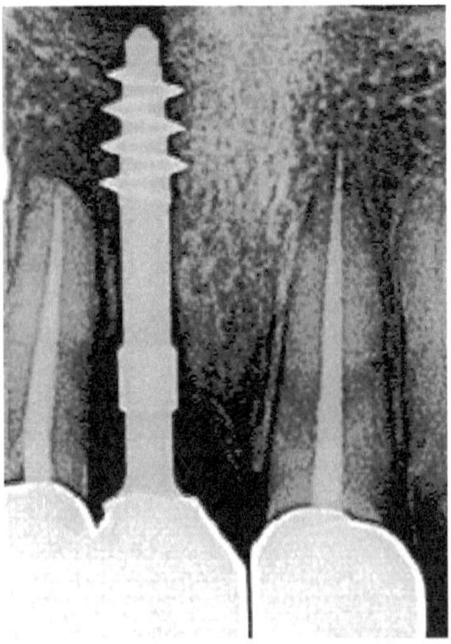

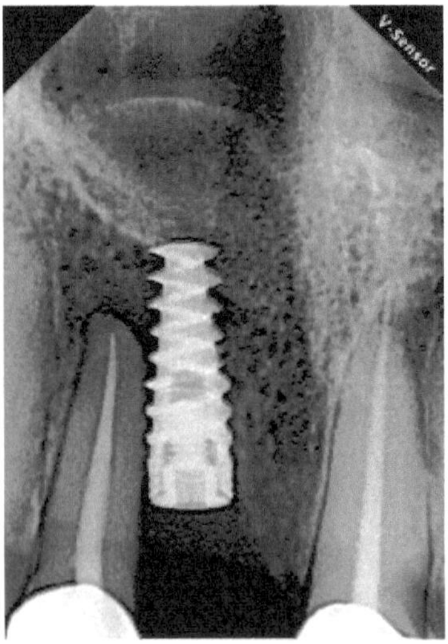

CHAPTER - 7

THE BASAL IMPLANT JEOPARDY - EPISODE 2 OF MANY

"Nothing in the world is worth having or worth doing unless it means effort, pain, difficulty" - Theodore Roosevelt.

Basal Implants, as I previously discussed in the previous chapter, are not FDA approved, and it is a crude treatment for their inability to get screw-retained crowns on top of them. An important aspect of an implant is the retrievability of the crown, which is never an option with a basal implant.

You may wonder why many practitioners do basal implants. These implants are usually thin, barely 2.8 to 3.0 mm in diameter and if in case of a full mouth implant, will require at least 12 to 16 instead of the 6 with a conventional implant. These cannot be digitally planned, and hence, freehand is done by doctors, and these are mostly practised by doctors who are limited by their surgical exposure. I have seen many orthodontists who specialise in braces and aligners place basal implants; this is because of the simple surgical skills, cheaper cost of implants and crowns, and patients who are okay with anything that costs less.

This story is of a lady patient aged 65 years, Mrs Mayuri* (Name Changed), who had full mouth basal implants with a fixed Cemented prosthesis using Metal Ceramic Crowns. She had 12 implants in her mouth, out of which 9 were completely mobile and infected, and the entire prosthesis was shaking.

Surgery was planned, and all her implants were removed. One of the implants had integrated well, so I decided against retrieving it completely since it might cause bigger bone loss than leaving it sleeping under the gums.

I placed All on Four implants in her lower arch and gave her an immediate screw-retained hybrid prosthesis, which, to this day, for the past 6 years, has been with no issues.

Basal Implant, yet again, is the issue here, and patients undergo treatments thinking it's cheap, but the issues and pain and expenditure that happen over the next few years are not worth having.

Moral of the Story:

Be it mouth Implants or Single Implants, avoid Basal Implants at all costs for a peaceful life.

Cheaper is not always the best option, especially with Dental Implants.

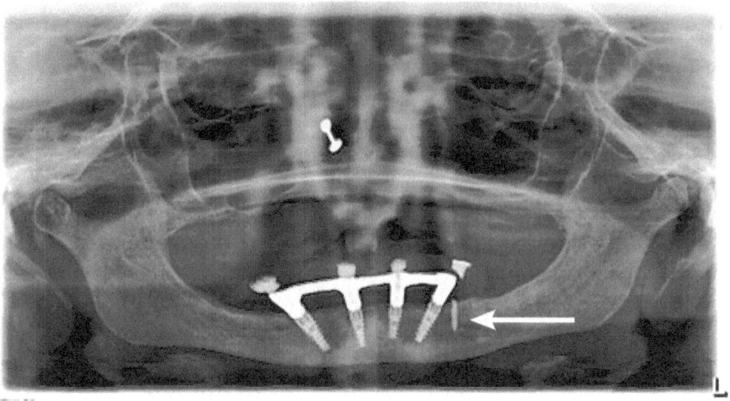

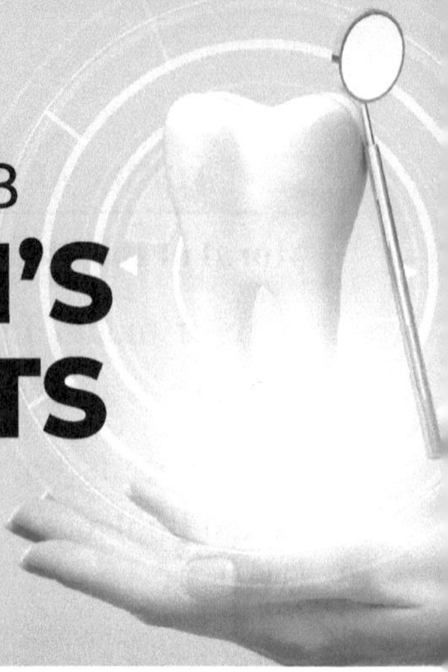

CHAPTER - 8
MY MOM'S IMPLANTS

"Jesus said to them, "A prophet is not without honour (respect) except in his hometown and among his relatives and in his own household."-Mark 6:4

Similarly, an Implantologist is respected everywhere for the work done except for with his relatives. This is a funny anecdote of me placing implants for my mother.

My mother is a retired teacher, who I know is the most famous teacher in my town. Whenever I go with her out in my town, at least 2 or 3 people come down to wish her and inform her that they are her students. I often jokingly mention that she should compete in elections and that she can easily win in any symbol and party owing to her popularity.

Dental disease also affected my mother, and she had her fair share of crowns, root canals and bridges done at my native place with different dentists. Her lower jaw showed a lot of teeth that were failing and were shaky.

Two years back, she decided to bite the bullet by getting treated with me. I remembered a scene from Vasoolraja

MBBS movie, where Prakash Raj, as a doctor, claims that his hands might shake if he operated on his daughter. I was also wondering if my hands would shake if I treated my mother.

My mother was a sweetheart during the surgery, and she later claimed proudly that I was the best dentist she had ever gotten treatment from. I had placed 6 implants in her lower jaw in a record 30-minute time. It was a free hand surgery, and yet, with careful CBCT studying, I was able to perform at that record speed. This, by far, is the fastest freehand 6 implants I have done in my career.

She recovered well, and a few crowns were immediately given to her. In 4 months, all the implants in her lower jaw were restored. The funny incident was during healing, my mother got annoyed with me on a particular day and, in anger, told me to remove all the RODS I installed in her jaw. I had to explain to her these were titanium medical devices and speak to her about how they get integrated into the bone. But she stuck with the term Iron Rod.

This apart, it was smooth sailing for her implants, even though she was diabetic with moderate control only. Recently, she mentioned to me that the teeth do not feel like a prosthesis and have become a part of her, and she has almost forgotten that she got implants, aka Rods, in her mouth. She eats well nowadays, and I have never been happier since I previously felt bad that I was restoring teeth for many patients who looked like my mother and had not treated my mother.

Now Happy Annachi!

Moral of the Story:

You may be however big, but for your parents and close relatives, you are still the little kid who played in the sand and built sand castles. Building bridges in the mouth using implants may still be nothing for them, yet they are your pillar of support. The family also always keeps you humble.

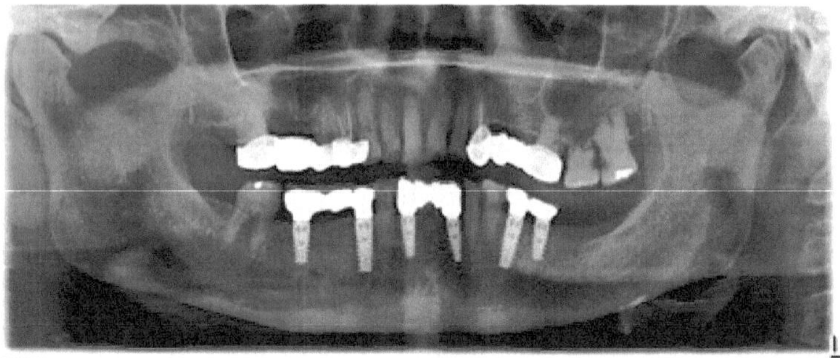

CHAPTER - 9

THE AIRHOSTESS CONUNDRUM

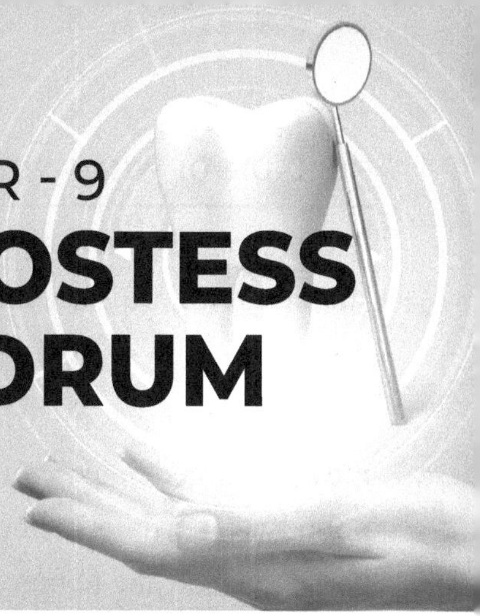

Having a dream from childhood is great. Achieving it in life is a dream come true. As a kid, I wanted to be in different professions at different phases of life, ranging from a Pilot to a Cardiologist.

I have always had a fantasy about flying, and this story is about a young girl who achieved her life ambition of being an air hostess.

Ms Caroline* (Name Changed), aged 23 years, was already a high-flying air hostess. She had travelled to over 25 countries at a young age and was with one of the premier airlines. She was a confident and self-reliant lady.

There, however, stood a small tooth between her and her career. She had a condition called Oligodontia or, in plain terms, a few missing permanent teeth. This doesn't mean she did not have gaps; rather, she had her milk tooth in her mouth. The missing tooth was her canine, which is the front tooth, and she still had her milk canine tooth in her mouth.

This milk tooth was designed to fall off when she was

9 years old, but it survived until 23, and unfortunately, it started giving way when she landed in London on one of the trips.

Her brother was my friend's employee, and they contacted me and wanted help in this regard. The tricky situation is that nobody can see her without teeth, and it may even cost her, her job, according to her. She was scared that her tooth might fall off anytime. She only had a window of 2 days in Chennai between two trips.

My team was ready, and by the time she landed at our clinic, we started working on her. The milk tooth was removed, and an immediate implant was placed in the canine region and in less than 30 minutes, she had her temporary tooth on it. There were no sutures, and I made sure the temporary crown pretty much looked like her previous milk tooth.

She went back really happy and came back again after 3 months to get her permanent screw-retained ceramic tooth.

It was a very satisfying case, and Caroline felt I had saved her job. But in reality, it was a simple, easy-peasy surgery and restoration. At times, little things that we do matter huge to others

Moral of the Story

Dreams shouldn't be shattered by Tooth loss. Dreams are bigger; keep dreaming and achieving. For the tooth, there are people like us. Nothing to worry.

CHAPTER - 10
THE SMOKING BELIEVER'S DOUBLE SINUS LIFT

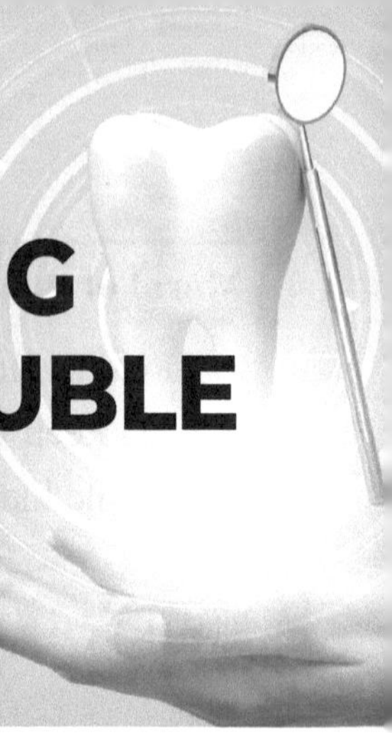

Smoking Kills! It does!

Smoking can also kill implants.

Smoking adversely affects Implant success. However, it is a relative contraindication and if the patient decides to stop smoking at least 3 weeks before implant surgery and 3 months after, then the success rate of the implant is predictable.

In 2013, I met a 50-year-old chain smoker, Mr Manokar*(Name Changed). He smokes a pack every day and is otherwise a very healthy man who does a lot of physical exercises.

He did not have his upper back teeth on both sides and if implants are to be done, a sinus lift will be warranted. Considering his smoking, I did not give him implants as my first choice. But the patient was very adamant. He wanted only implants.

I was very sceptical. But the patient was super insistent on getting implants. The words he used to convince me were that he believed in me and knew that my surgical skills would counter any issues caused by smoking. He was a super believer.

I told him to avoid smoking for 3 weeks, and I was told he stopped smoking, but I doubt it though. The surgeries went smoothly with direct sinus lifting and implants on both sides and after healing of close to 6 months, I gave him screw-retained zirconia crowns.

It was amazing to note the healing went uneventful and, at times, beliefs do work. Even then, I did advise him to stop smoking for all its ill effects on the body. Very recently, he did a 10-year review, and his implants and crowns were put with not a single millimetre of bone loss.

It was an amazing story where the patient believed in me more than me! It was the last case where I did a Sinus lift on a chronic smoker, and I may not do that anymore, though.

Moral of the Story

Positivity and Belief keep us running. However, blind faiths are discouraged.

And definitely, Smoking is Injurious.

If You need dental implants, quit smoking.

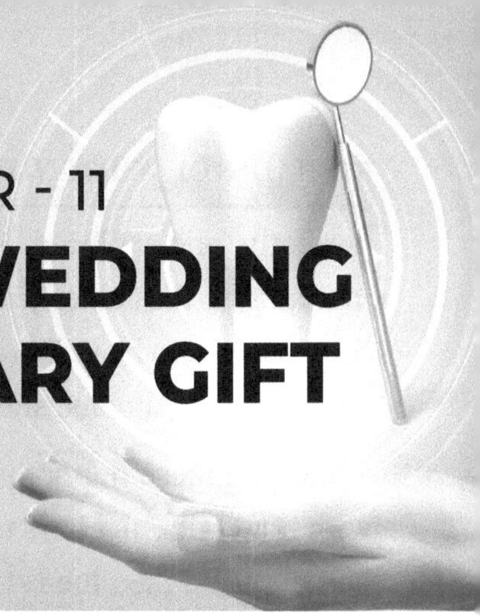

CHAPTER - 11
THE BEST WEDDING ANNIVERSARY GIFT

Some people touch your lives when you touch their lives. Some people become fans of your work. Some people become Brand Ambassadors for you. Then, there are some people who are all of the above.

This is a heart-touching story of a 41-year-old female, Lakshmi* (Name Changed). I vividly remember the day I met her. She was this lady with no front teeth in the upper and lower arches and was wearing a removable partial denture or a flipper, which she got done when she was in London*(City Changed). She has been wearing this for quite some time, and many doctors she met had advised her against implants since she had a very thin bone.

In my first consult, when I told her of a treatment plan where I could place implants, she cried sitting in the dental chair. At that time, I did not know the magnitude of her suffering all these years.

I decided to split the bone in the upper jaw and graft the jaw along with the placement of the implant. The split went perfectly, and I placed 3 implants in the upper jaw and 2 implants in the lower jaw and left the implants submerged for 6 months to heal. During this time, she continued to wear her denture and made sure the wound healed satisfactorily.

During these 6 months, Lakshmi and her husband, along with her children, come for reviews, and I have seldom seen her talk. And then the D day happened. The delivery of final teeth.

I gave her fixed Zirconia teeth over her upper and lower front teeth, and they were perfect. And it was time to throw her dentures away for good. I could see the level of confidence that suddenly popped into her eyes after fixed permanent teeth were given to her. I also learnt that the day I delivered her final prosthesis was on her wedding Anniversary. She was so happy that she got her best gift ever: a new smile and confidence.

After this, her transformation was phenomenal. I learnt that she was a voracious extrovert and that she liked to talk about loads of stuff. She also did complete research on me, such as where I studied and about my family members, etc. I even joked that she should take up a job as an online detective vetting employees or wannabe brides and bridegrooms.

Her daughter and son gifted me customised gifts, and they follow my every move in YouTube videos.

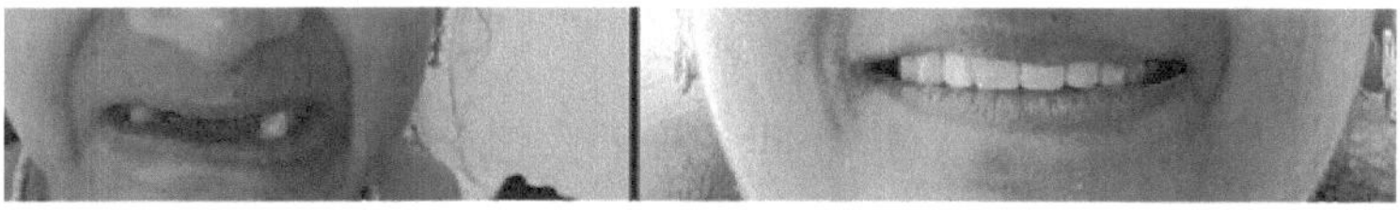

Recently, again, I had called her for a 1.5-year review on a particular day, not knowing it was her birthday. After the review, I felt really bad that I made her come to the Clinic on her birthday instead of visiting a Temple. She immediately replied that the clinic was her temple since all her problems were solved there. I was at a loss of words hearing this.

We celebrated her birthday with her family in our clinic, and this patient has become a friend and her family a family for me and my staff.

It was one of the most emotional stories for me in my career.

Moral of the Story

Earning money is the easiest part of life. Earning people is the toughest part.

My profession lets me earn people by doing my job.

Earn people! Earn Happiness! And God Bless!

CHAPTER - 12

MARRIAGES FIXED AFTER DENTAL IMPLANTS

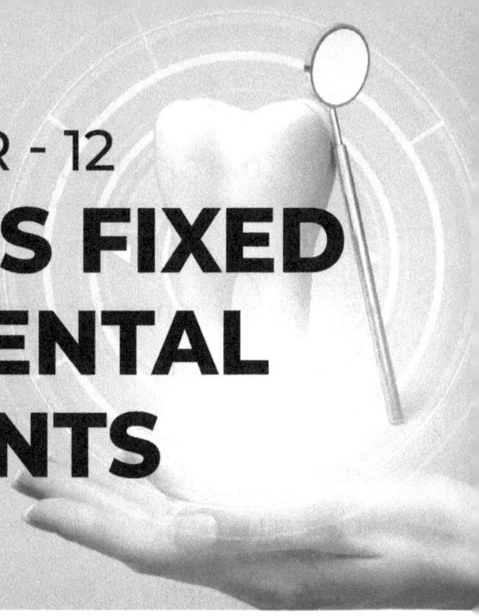

They say Marriages are fixed in Heaven! But we can also claim a few marriages are fixed due to Dental Clinics. These are 2 stories of young people who were finding it difficult to get the knot tied.

There is a situation called Aggressive Periodontitis. This is an aggressive form of gum disease where certain teeth are lost very early, or most of the teeth become shaky, and patients find it difficult to eat and function. The most problematic thing with aggressive periodontitis is that the teeth move outward, and there will be conspicuous proclined and gap-filled teeth. Also, halitosis (Bad smell from the mouth) is deplorable.

This story is of my youngest Aggressive Periodontitis patient, Bhuvaneswari* (Name Changed), who lost all her teeth when she was 21 years old. She was depressed all the way, and I vividly remember her mother crying to me. This was 2009 days, and I had placed more than 6 implants in her upper jaw and 6 implants in her lower and restored her smile in about 3 months.

What I remember from this patient was that, while she had temporaries on, she told me that she got engaged and her marriage fixed after the permanent teeth. Gave me the utmost happiness of the way dental implants touched and changed somebody's life.

A year later, I happened to meet her with her husband, and the guy was thankful enough to me, and he even got one molar implant in his mouth later.

Couples that get Implants together! Stay Together!

The second story is of a 34-year-old Software Engineer named Arun* (Name Changed), who is incidentally from my native place, the southernmost tip of India, Kanyakumari. He found me over the internet and came with extremely bad dentition, abused over the years. One distinctive trait that I noted with him was that he was always shy and seemed very introverted. I also learned he had multiple proposals rejected owing to his bad teeth and bad smell.

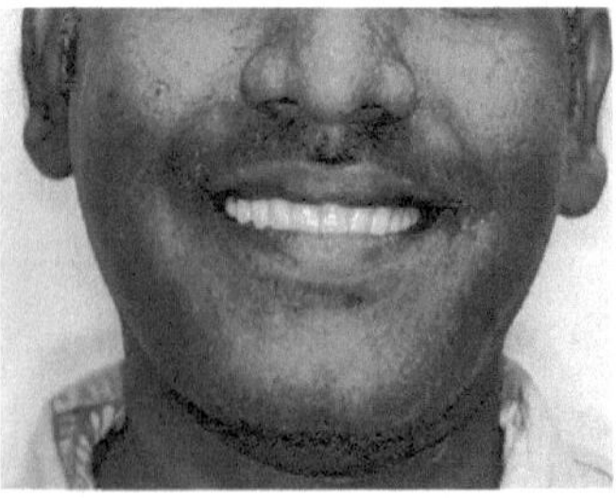

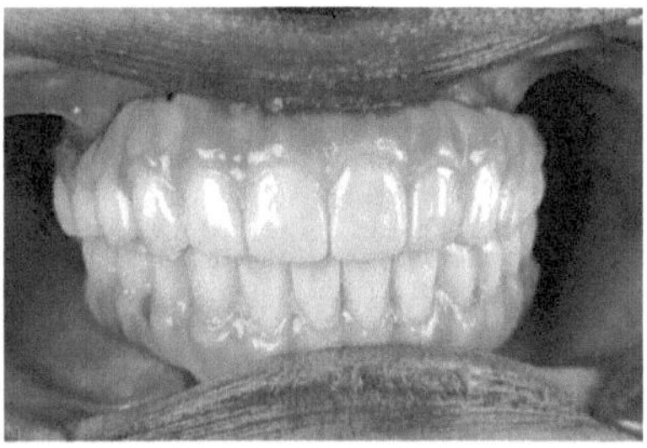

It was decided to let go of all teeth and place full-mouth implants, and he got his final teeth in 3 months, which were mouth Zirconia teeth. During one of the visits, he told me he got engaged to a Nurse from Saudi Arabia and their marriage was fixed in the latter half of the year. He was ecstatic, and after his permanent teeth, I could see a more confident and happy individual. Both the stories are spaced at least 14 years, a lifetime in fact; however, they have the same storyline with two youngsters suffering because of aggressive periodontitis.

Moral of The Story

Tooth Loss can happen even at a young age. Intervene early with simple procedures, which can save a lot of money and issues in later life. A Dentist visit, at times, saves lives and, at times, also money.

Happiness cannot be bought; however, having a good Implantologist can also bring happiness.

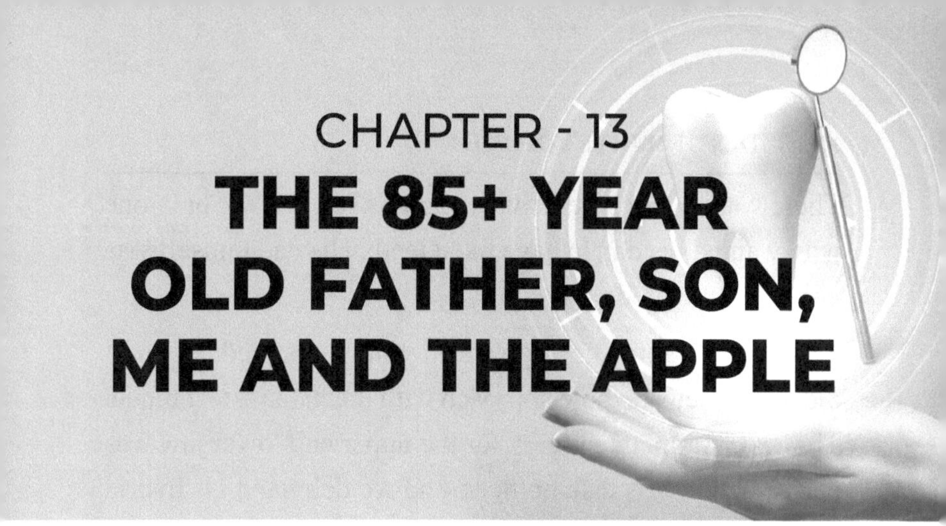

CHAPTER - 13
THE 85+ YEAR OLD FATHER, SON, ME AND THE APPLE

"Fathering is not something perfect men do, but something that perfects men." - Frank Pittman. My father is my superhero, and I have tried to be a superhero to my daughter. Being a father is easy as your child grows older.

However, as Parents age, Children become Parent-like and take care of their Parents. That is the reason why old age is also called second childhood. And in second childhood, people lose most of their teeth to disease.

This is the story of an 85-plus-year-old father and his son. The father definitely is older than 85 years, and nobody knows his exact age. His last son, who is 45 years visited me along with his father. His father had lost all his teeth 20 years back. He had tried some dentures, but he never liked any and never used any.

His son wanted to improve his father's nutrition by giving him new teeth. The story also involves his 5 elder brothers and sisters, who were against any sort of surgery for him.

There was so much negativity, and this son was the only one who wanted his dad to have fixed teeth. His dad himself was not that motivated.

The son wanted us to go ahead with the procedure, and I did a complete keyhole approach with the flapless technique. The whole implant surgery for the upper and lower jaw was performed in less than an hour, and we delivered his hybrid prosthesis in less than a week.

The entire family was very happy to see their father with teeth. One week progressed, and the father came back to me with a complaint. When he never had teeth, he had the habit of twisting his tongue constantly. Now that he had fixed teeth, the tongue felt as if it was in prison and could not move everywhere like it could when he had no teeth. He also was not chewing his food and was swallowing it without teeth. A habit for over 20 years cannot be changed immediately in a week.

I started doing my usual counselling, where I taught him to use his teeth to chew. A second childhood with teething issues! The son was so happy when I made his father eat an apple in front of him. Yes, now he could eat an apple; it was just that it needed a little practice.

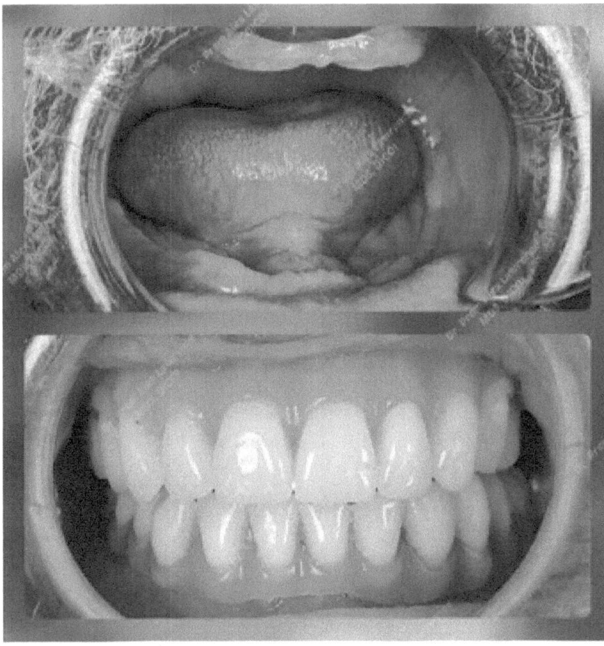

Now, after 6 months, I hear the son tell me that his father is eating better and is now eating hard foods that he has never had in over 20 years. The son is also constantly counselling his father to chew better. The son's effort to get his father a better dentition, not just spending money but being there throughout the process, was commendable.

Moral of the Story:

If your parents still call you over the phone or in person, you are lucky to have them. Serve them the best of the life and treat them with respect.

A good dentition is the simplest gift that you can offer your parent in their old age. Get their blessings always! And stay with them in their difficult times. Our children would also treat us the same way we treat our parents.

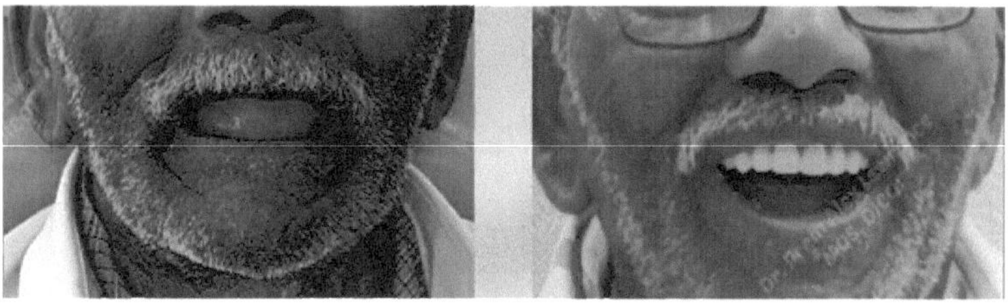

CHAPTER - 14

THE YOGA TEACHER WHO WAS SCARED OF INJECTIONS

I once told my patient that I can give "Painless Injections". My patient asked me back that the Injection itself is painful; how can it be painless? I laughed all the way when the patient made me understand it was an oxymoron.

This is the story of a Yoga Teacher of about 45 years who was so scared of visiting a dentist, let alone an Implantologist. She made a call to my office in 2021 and wanted to know if Implants could be placed in a painless process, but she also did not want sedation or general anaesthesia. She was scared of any sort of injections.

She wanted to know if anaesthesia could be given just by inhalation and not with injections. When explained that only a sedative given as an injection in her hand would make her sleep and after that, all implants could be placed, she took one year to decide on this.

In 2022, She decided to take the plunge. She was so scared before surgery that, for some reason, it was the toughest case that I performed with my anaesthetist, Dr Navaneetha

Krishnan. She was somehow keeping herself awake and asked the anaesthetist for more drugs to doze her off. It may be some yogic way of resisting sedation.

Her bone was so bad that I had to literally search for bone to place all her implants and do a lot of bone grafting. She was made to wait for 6 weeks before a definitive prosthesis was made. She went back happy, and her dental issue was sorted like never before.

I recently met her for a one-year review where, again, she was scared that I might give her an injection. I understood that her fear of injection came from her childhood times when she got painful extractions done.

She is now happy, and she has a place for rental in her home where she wants me to set up an implant clinic. It was a sweet gesture when she offered that.

Moral of the Story

Being scared of needles is a true phobia. But modern dentistry has grown manifolds where thinner needles and painless injections are the order of the day. Sleep Dentistry is used alongside many major dental procedures, which are extremely safe and effective when such a phobia exists.

Dentist Offices are not scary anymore!

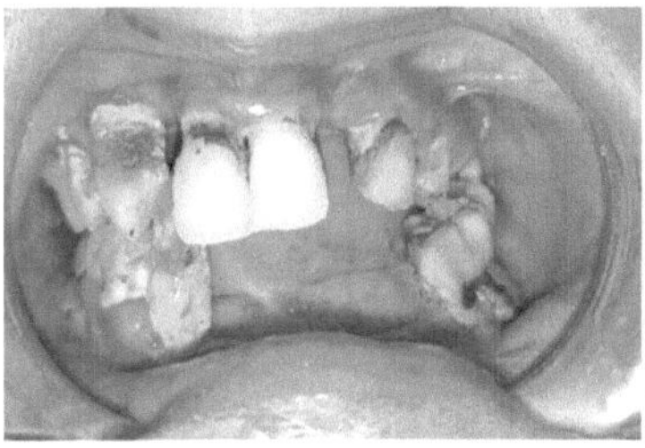

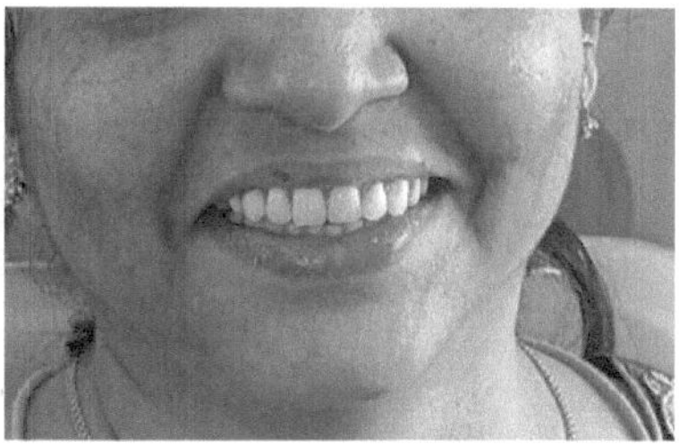

CHAPTER - 15

THE CANCER SURVIVOR AND HER IMPLANTS

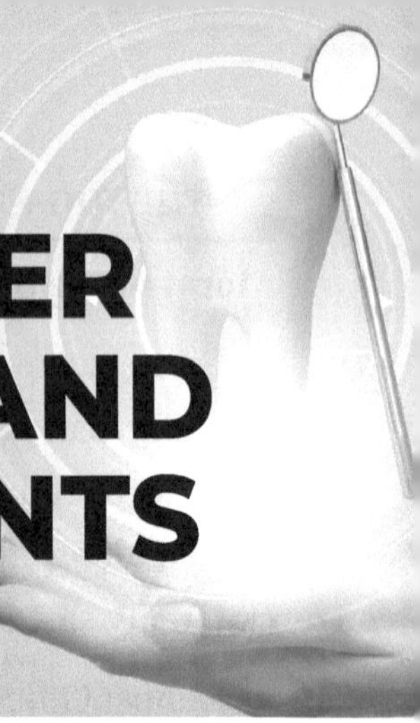

"You can be a victim of Cancer or a survivor of Cancer. It's a Mindset" - Dave Pelzer

Cancer is never the end of life. We hear a multitude of stories of strength, valour and win. Once they win Cancer, many issues around the dentition need to be attended to. If radiation is done, it usually results in less saliva in the mouth, resulting in increased dental decay and other oral diseases.

Menaka* (Name Changed) was a Breast Cancer survivor. She was devastated when she learned that she was having this disease. When she recovered, she had more devastation than when she had lost her husband. The first time I met her, she was all in tears and tatters.

Her sons wanted good teeth for her, and she never talked to me all through the treatment time. I decided on full mouth rehabilitation owing to her decay in almost all her teeth and mobile teeth as well. I performed Four Implants in both jaws and gave her an immediate hybrid prosthesis.

She never reacted much when her prosthesis was fixed. But the thing changed when she came for the one-week review. Her usual sorrow face was not there. She was happy that she was able to eat into everything, and her usual proclined teeth were replaced by better-looking, better-functioning teeth.

Recently, I met her for a 6-month review. She had a minor ulcer for which I removed her lower prosthesis for 3 days when she completely opened up to me that she was able to eat everything, and she had also gained some weight post this treatment. She told me that her prosthesis doesn't feel different and is now a part of her.

Her ulcer healed, and I gave back HER tooth after 4 days. She is happier than ever.

Moral of The Story

Cancer is never the end, and Time heals any wound, and we can move on from anything. All it needs is good mental strength and strong support from family and friends. All the side effects of cancer therapy can be handled easily.

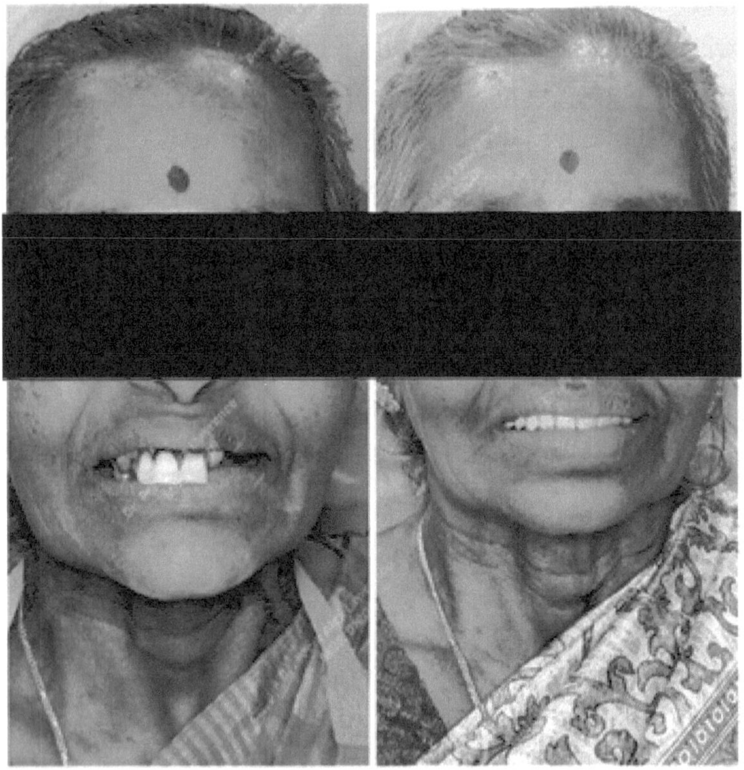

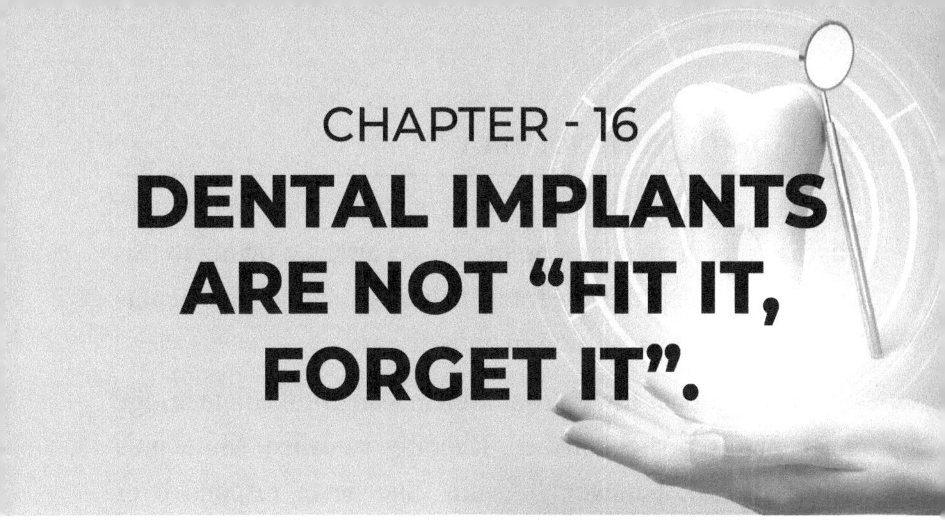

CHAPTER - 16

DENTAL IMPLANTS ARE NOT "FIT IT, FORGET IT".

Many patients think any dental treatment, once done, lasts a lifetime, and there is no need to visit the dentist or surgeon for the particular problem in their lives again. Especially for implant patients, if they miss the maintenance appointments, there is a chance of minor issues becoming bigger.

I have had patients who vanish completely and never come in touch with the doctor. The majority of patients' mindsets are the same. Unless the patient gets some issue, they never visit a doctor. I have an automated system which reminds all my patients about a year's review, and also, they are personally wished on their birthday.

This story is about a patient who missed her reviews for 6 years, and then, when an issue happened, she searched and found me on the Internet and visited to get it corrected.

In 2017, a 50-year-old female patient named Janaki* (Name Changed) had lower front teeth, which were shaky, and came to me for a solution. The lower front teeth have the shortest and most slender roots in the oral cavity. When gum disease sets in, they are the first to get affected owing to this and also because the lower teeth always accumulate calculus in the back side, resulting in gum disease.

Janaki got her lower front implants and immediate bridge in them. Then she vanished. Literally vanished. My team's efforts to call her went in vain. She never responded or ignored our calls.

However, very recently, in 2023, she found my contact information from Google and Practo and contacted us. The reason, she had a minor gum enlargement around the implants, and some doctors had a differential diagnosis of oral cancer.

Janaki at last visited me. On examination, I could see a lot of tartar under the bridge, which probably would not have been cleaned for more than 5 years. This tartar had irritated the gums and caused a hyperplasia (benign growth). I immediately removed the bridge from the implant since they were screw-retained and excised the growth with soft tissue LASER.

Janaki healed uneventfully, and the bridge was placed back, she committed to visiting me once a year and not, only during any issues.

Moral of the Story:

Implants are Not "Fit it and Forget it Devices". I always tell my patients the analogy of owning a car. You will have to get it serviced once in a while. Similarly, Implants need a check-up once a year, which will avoid heartbreaks later in life.

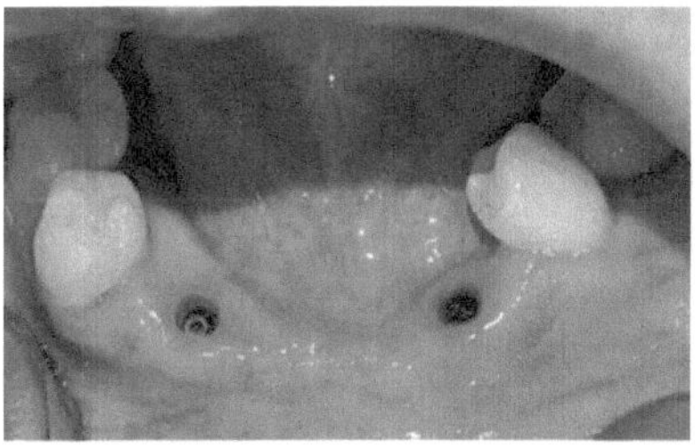

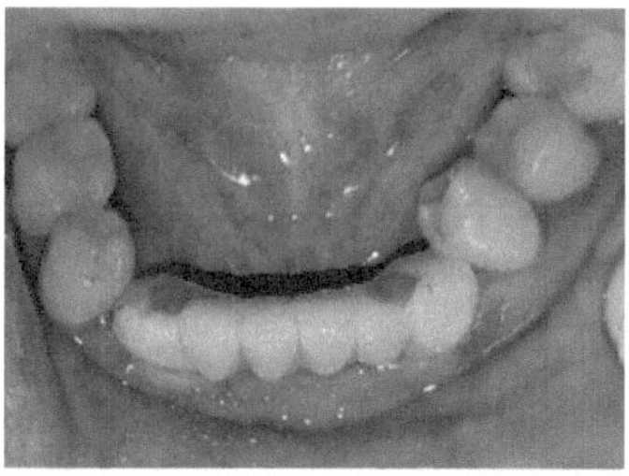

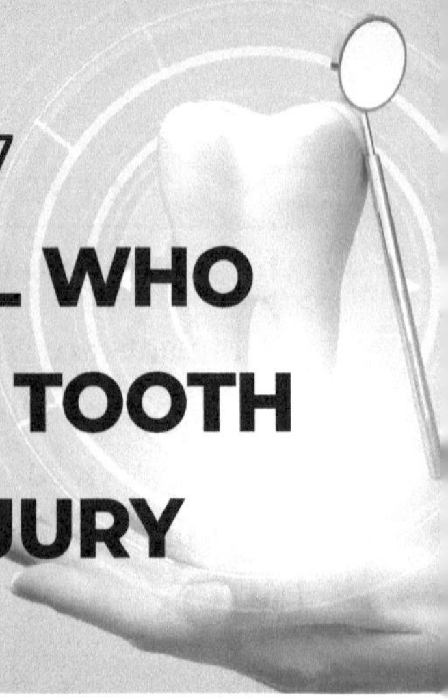

CHAPTER - 17

THE YOUNG GIRL WHO LOST HER FRONT TOOTH TO SPORTS INJURY

Studies say that 5 million people lose a tooth resulting from sports-related accidents per year, and 50% of children playing sports face a dental injury before they complete school. Though this data is for the American population, I guess the percentage should be way higher in the Indian population. I remember during my school days, at least ten such incidents involving my classmates where a tooth was injured.

This story is about a young girl of age 21 years named Sheethal* (Name Changed) from Lucknow* (City Changed) who works in a software company in Chennai and comes to me with a unique problem. She had a sports injury where her front tooth got hurt in childhood and got discoloured over some time. She also started developing infections around that tooth, which caused much pain and swelling.

She had gotten root canal treatments multiple times in the tooth, and most of the time, it did not last for over a year, and she had to suffer for a long time. The tooth had failed and had resorbed roots and infection when she visited me.

I had a precarious situation. This was a young girl's front tooth. And it was hugely infected. With the CBCT scan, I knew there was a huge defect in the outer aspect of the bone. It was like. Literally, I needed to build one wall of the room, which was broken down completely without disturbing the other walls.

When a tooth is removed, the gums and the bone go for a toss as soon as 5 minutes, and the lost bone and time cannot be recovered. Hence, I had to be swift in this case.

I carefully extracted the tooth, and when I opened her gums, I saw a huge defect. I placed a good Nobel Active Ti-ultra ® implant in the extracted site. After cleaning it, I started building the wall with artificial bone and a membrane and closed the site to make sure maximum bone was preserved.

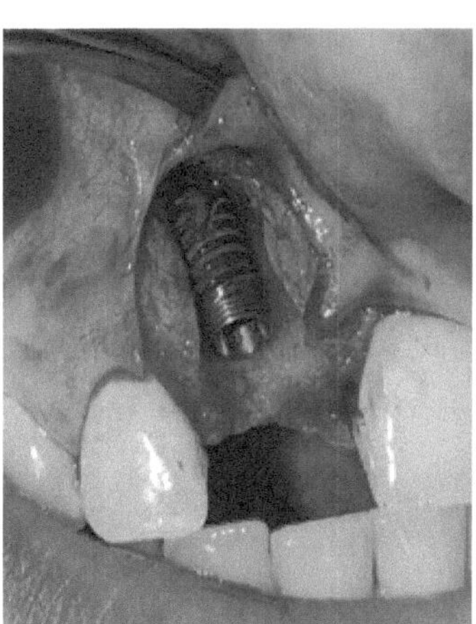

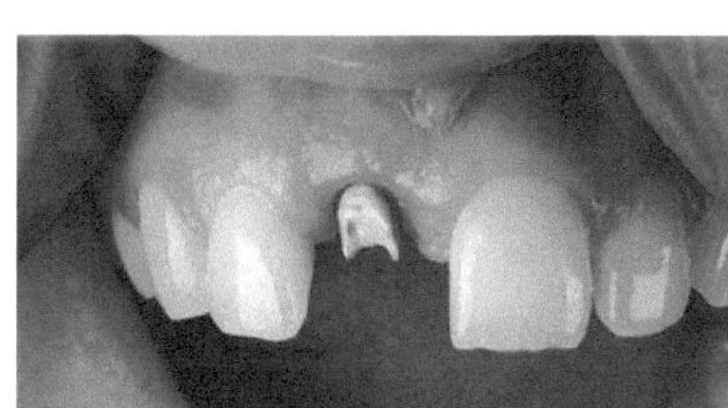

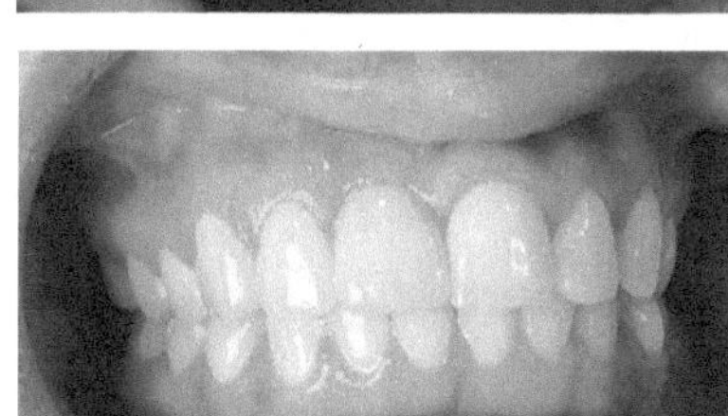

We allowed it to heal for about 5 months, and Sheethal was so cooperative that she would visit me even when she had some minor doubts about healing. A major amount of time was spent on selecting Sheethal's tooth colour since she had a very unique shade. Finally, we decided on the shade, and a very good-looking crown was given, preserving the bone and gums and also regenerating the bone wherever required.

Sheethal's patience was commendable in this case, and I, too, felt this was one case where my surgical skills were used in full.

Moral of the Story:

Often, a mild discoloured front tooth due to some minor injury may fail at a later stage. If it fails and warrants Implants, it requires specialized skill to regrow bone clear infections and restore the tooth.

Stained and Discoloured Front teeth are bad. Get them rectified.

Play Sports! But protect your teeth!

CHAPTER - 18
"THE FOOT IN THE DOOR" IMPLANT TREATMENT

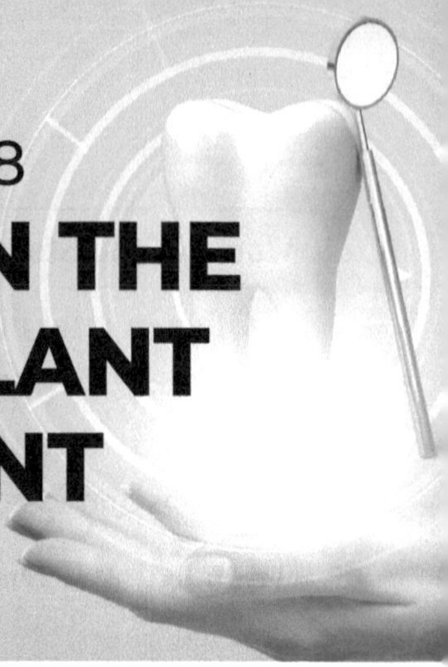

In businesses, the foot-in-the-door technique is when a small request is initially made in order to get a person to agree to a bigger request later. In dentistry, doctors resort to the foot-in-the-door technique many times.

This is the story of a 65-year-old man who was in a senior position in a multinational corporation. He travels a lot and is often out of India for years. He came to me with a problem of gum disease and shaky teeth and wanted a permanent solution. But all that he could give me was only 4 days. He was a diabetic as well, and his diabetes was very well within control.

He had exhaustively researched Dental Implants with Dr Google and Dr Internet. He had come up with his own treatment plan.

After examining him, I found that he needed full-mouth rehabilitation and full-mouth implants. But the time he gave me was limited; hence, he wanted a fix of just the lower front teeth. I was obliged to do that, and I placed two implants in the lower front region and gave him immediate final teeth.

Since he will be abroad for a whole year, I told him that the next time he goes to India, he will add 4 more implants in his lower arch and give fully fixed teeth. Though I may not be obliged to do such part treatments, I had to agree with this gentleman since he was in a rush and in a high position where he needed a solution immediately.

I call this the "Foot in the Door, rather than Mouth" treatment.

Moral of the Story:

Dr Google is not the best doctor in town. The Internet provides information that is not always reliable. For a basic understanding, Dr Google is good. To deep dive, you need a physical doctor.

Foot-the-door technique in Implant planning is not harmful if the patient gets the rest of the treatment in a fixed time frame.

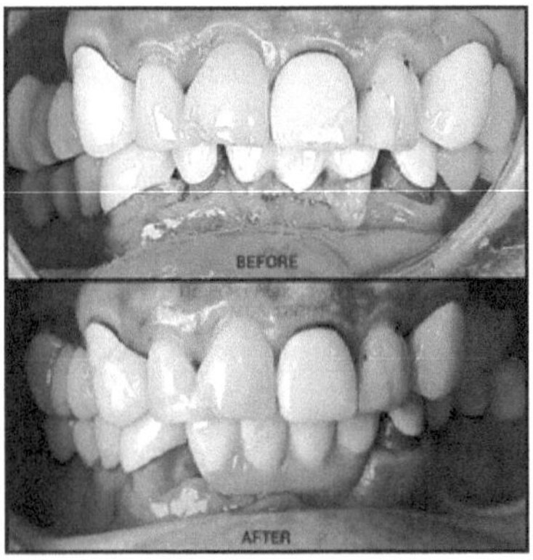

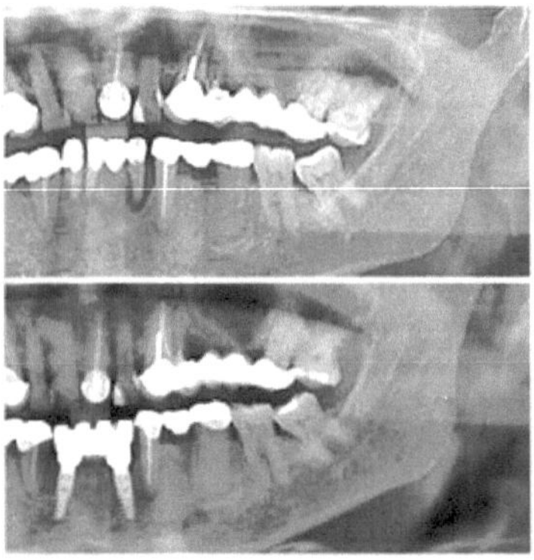

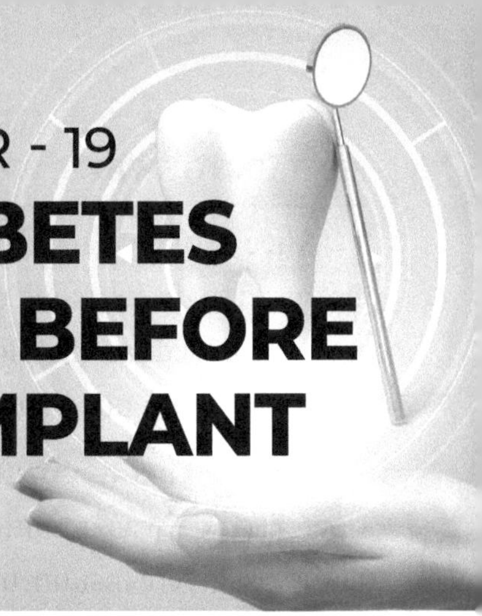

CHAPTER - 19
THE DIABETES DISCOVERY BEFORE DENTAL IMPLANT

Diabetes is a deadly disease. Often, it is a silent killer. Many Diabetic individuals do not know they are diabetic and walk around with the disease. Personally, I have diagnosed diabetes for multitudes of patients with gum problems.

The story starts in Canada*(Country Changed). A 52-year-old lady named Alice* (Name Changed) wanted to get full mouth implants with me since all her teeth were shaky and infected. We had an online consultation done, where it was revealed that she was never diabetic. With a CBCT scan done in Canada, we did a treatment plan involving Six Implants and Zirconia Teeth. I had requested her to block 6 weeks of time to get the entire treatment done.

She happily arrived in Chennai, and my Facility Manager, Venu, picked her and her sons up from the airport and brought them to a Hotel near my premises. The same day, when we took a routine blood picture, she got the shock of her life that she was diabetic.

Alice was devastated, but she wanted the dental treatment. I refused to do Implants with such high sugar levels. We had to work to reduce the blood sugar level as soon as possible since she could not change her travel plans.

I referred her to my good friend Dr Rajeswari, a medical doctor. Alice was admitted to the Hospital of Dr Rajeswari and was given insulin treatment over a period of 10 days admission when her sugar level was brought under control.

After getting medical fitness, my team and I proceeded with implant placement under a controlled environment and avoided any major trauma. Luckily, her bone quality and quantity were very good, so we could get good Primary stability on the implant, and I proceeded with permanent crown placement immediately. Her blood sugar was monitored constantly, and she was advised to keep it in check for the next 3 months and also for the rest of her life.

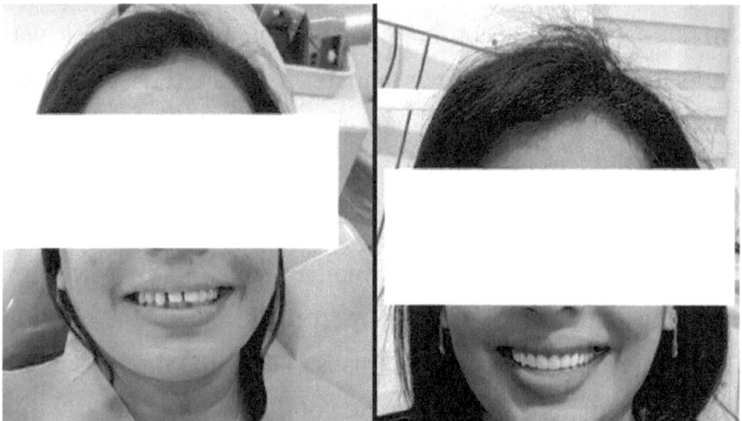

She diligently followed everything, and once crowns were given, she was extremely happy that she sent her children to Canada early. She wanted to spend a week in Chennai and Pondicherry to party and go shopping.

Though I had to work with an unexpectedly shortened time limit, this was a very satisfactory case where, again, my surgical skills were best used.

Moral of The Story

Diabetes is Deadly. It's rather unlucky when somebody becomes diabetic. A hormone called Insulin, which gets abused by people when it is not sufficiently secreted, creates all sorts of issues in the body and affects every organ.

Respect Insulin when you have it! But Diabetes, again, is not the end of the road, too!

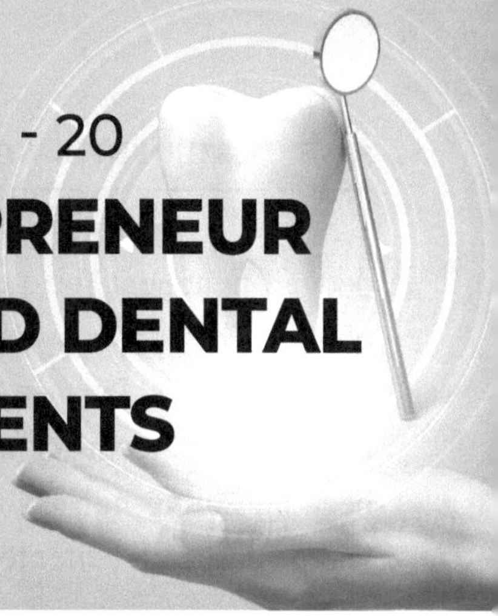

CHAPTER - 20

THE ENTREPRENEUR WHO DODGED DENTAL TREATMENTS

Health is the last thing that any entrepreneur has in his or her mind. I also fall into the same category. Health is often neglected, and Dental or Oral health is never a priority at all.

This story happened during peak COVID days. The story is about a 54-year-old man, Williams*(Name Changed), who happens to own multiple retail shops spread across Chennai. One of my friends, Dr Xavier, an Orthodontist, referred him to me. Dr Xavier knew he had gum disease and wanted me to have a look at Williams.

Williams had fairly good oral health, except for his lower front teeth. These teeth were shaky and were non-salvageable. But Williams had other plans.

He could not come to the fact that his teeth were bad and thought he could live with it. But they were shaky to an extreme level. Fast forward 6 months. I saw him arrive at my office to get treatment, as I suggested.

I was wondering how a busy guy like him, who had dodged treatment for quite some time, decided to take the plunge. The answer was simple. He pointed it out to one of my doctors, Dr Jananee, who kept reminding him of the ill effects of his teeth for the past 6 months. Dr Jananee had been educating him behind the curtain and convinced him that he deserved better teeth.

The surgery went simply like any lower anterior implant surgery. The healing was good. We gave him an immediate temporary bridge and, after 6 weeks, a final Zirconia bridge.

While in review appointments, he kept lamenting the time lost when he was not decided and felt that he could have had better teeth early if he had listened to me, Dr Jananee and Dr Xavier at that time.

Moral of the Story:

Always take the plunge if you have decided. Delaying any decision in life changes a lot of metrics, and it may not be the same at a later date.

Fortunately, in Implant dentistry, a little delay is fine. But a larger delay will put you in a difficult situation and may be heavy on your pockets as well.

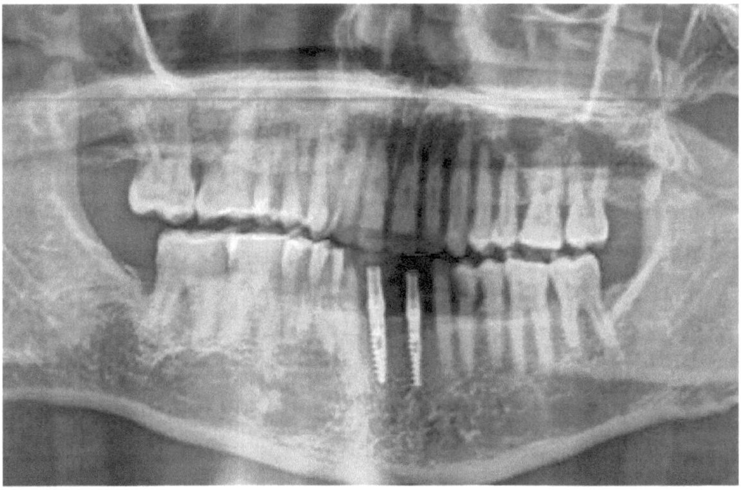

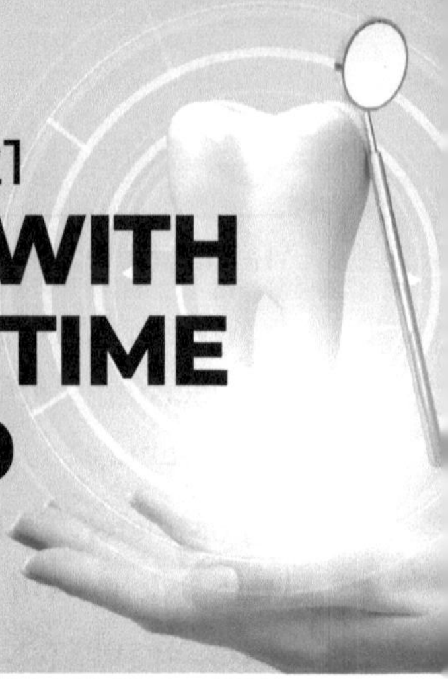

CHAPTER - 21

THE SAILOR WITH HIS LIMITED TIME IN LAND

Being a sailor is one of the toughest jobs in the world. Going to sea may be enchanting for most of us, but for the sailors who live most of their lives surrounded by water, land is heaven. The important thing is that access to medical health care is very limited in the sea. To see a doctor or dentist, they need to wait for months.

I met this Sailor recently who had moderate Aggressive Periodontitis (An aggressive form of Gum Disease), and he told me that he would be on land for the next month and then for 10 months, he would be back to the sea. He had tooth pain and abscesses, and on the ship, he could only get access to painkillers. He had been doing this for months, and the moment he landed, he came to meet me.

On examination, I could see multiple issues. However, we decided to attend to a few highly problematic issues since we were working with a time limit. We also had to ensure he did not have any issues while on the sea.

I performed a direct sinus lift on either side and placed 3 implants in the upper jaw and 2 implants in the lower front teeth, which were replaced immediately with a temporary bridge. I worked in the time we got. This was only possible with my in-house Laboratory and skilled technicians. He has now left for sea and should be back in 10 months for his permanent teeth.

Time on Land is like Gold for many professionals. Sailors deserve all the salute!

Moral of the Story:

There are two rules in any Profession:

Rule No.1: Understand the needs of each Client. They may not have all the time in the world. Respect that. Work accordingly

Rule No.2: Follow Rule No.1

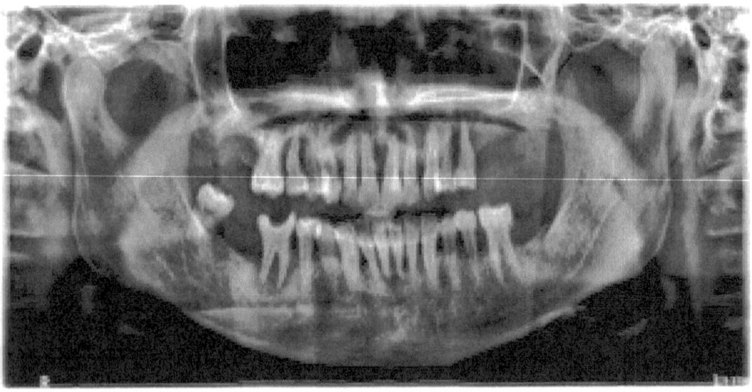

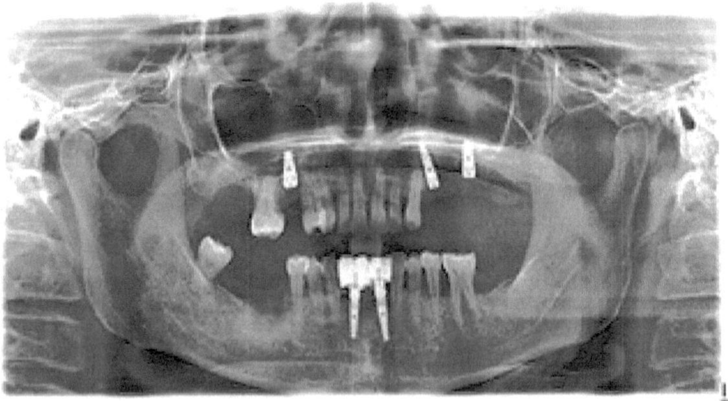

CHAPTER - 22

"SHE IS MY MOM" - MY NURSE MRS CHITRA'S STORY

A team does not succeed without its members. I often tell my team that we all are one cogwheel of a big machine, and if one wheel doesn't work, the machine does not do its job effectively. My team has been a well-oiled machine, with each player knowing their roles and responsibilities to full effect. From my security officer, Mr Mani, to me, we know what our role is as a wheel in our machine.

I will be indebted if I don't talk about my Implant Nurse, Mrs Chitra's story here. She has been with me since 2012, and in most of my career implant cases, she has stood beside me as my assistant. She knows exactly what material or equipment I will use next, and even before I want it, she is ready with it. She has also made sure the rest of my team, which includes Ms Bharathi, Mrs Banu, Mrs Meenakshi and others, are trained and ready to handle not just cases but also me. Today, I can proudly declare that Chitra knows Implant dentistry better than many undergraduate doctors.

This story is about an implant patient whom I treated 2 years back. A 60-year-old female patient named Kiran* (Name Changed), a high-profile patient, had a few missing teeth since childhood. Her native is Manipur, and she was married to a Tamilian. She had very bad experiences in her childhood with dental issues there. Hence, she was extremely scared of getting any dental treatment.

She met me, and she was convinced to get her treatment done with me. The only issue was she never wanted any injection. Hence, we decided to do it under conscious sedation.

The surgery went fine with sleep dentistry. Kiran was extremely comfortable during the 2-hour procedure. Usually, all patients do not remember anything that happened during the sedation, and once the procedure is done, the drug is withdrawn, and patients come to consciousness.

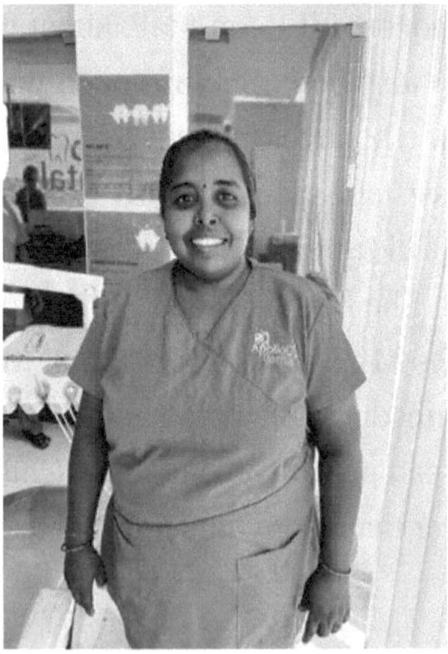

Usually, since this procedure is done with fasting for about 4 hours, once the procedure is done, we advise the attendee to get ice cream and feed the patient. However, with most patients, it is Chitra who feeds them. In this case, too, Chitra fed Kiran ice cream mixed with a painkiller.

The patient was so moved with emotions that she started calling Chithra her MOM. The reason was that the last time somebody fed food to her was her mom, and she fondly remembered her mother. She also called Chithra her second mom.

These were such moving scenes in the post-operative area of our surgical room, and I thought that Kiran was talking so under the mild influence of drugs. However, when she came again for review the next week for the removal of stitches, she remembered Chitra and called her mom again.

This is one of the many stories in which Chitra plays centre stage. She does connect with all the patients with simple humbleness and simpleness, which is a trait each one of us can follow.

Moral of the Story:

It is not every day we work with passion and ownership. Wherever we work, if we can have ownership of the job, we become the vital cog wheel in the running of the machine called Organisation.

Take ownership. Stay humble. Be like Chitra!

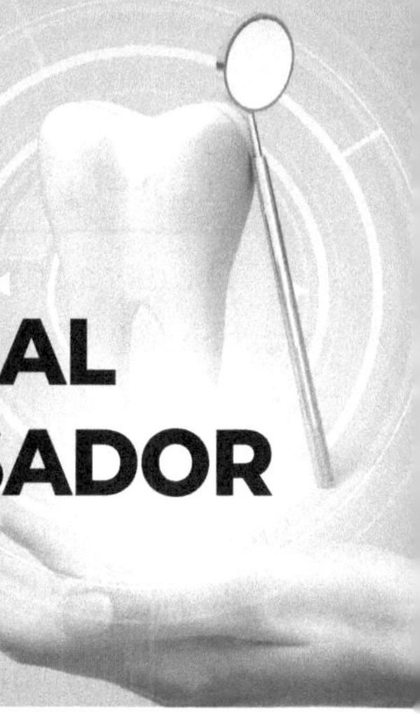

CHAPTER - 23
MY PERPETUAL BRAND AMBASSADOR

This should have been the 1st Chapter of this book. I used to tell my friends that I would have to write a book to write about this guy in my life.

He was one of my earliest implant patients in 2005. His name is Gopal*(Name Changed). He represents all of the Millennials as well as Generation Z. One fine day, out of nowhere, he ended up in my clinic with a missing tooth. His upper right premolar was missing, and I placed an implant with an immediate crown. That was just the start of my association with him.

The funny thing is I would have met him only about 5 times in these 18 years, but he keeps connecting with me somehow. Post-implant, he had to get 3 root canal treatments, too. I also fixed an appointment with my endodontist, a root canal specialist. Gopal wanted the appointment at 9 am since he worked night shifts and wanted to get the treatment done after his shift.

The day arrived, and the doctor was here, but Gopal never responded. We waited for 4 hours calling him, but he never picked up. At last, at 6 pm, he called me to apologize and say that he had overslept. He rescheduled the appointment for another day. Another day, same story. He sleeps, and we wait.

The funny thing was, as it happened the third time, we decided we would not block the appointment again unless he walked into the clinic. The fourth time was a charm; he came, got his root canals done and got his crown done with similar episodes.

He was one of my worst complying patients. Though I advised him to stop smoking after the implants, he never did. He is such a pain as a patient but has been an advocate for me for the past 18 years.

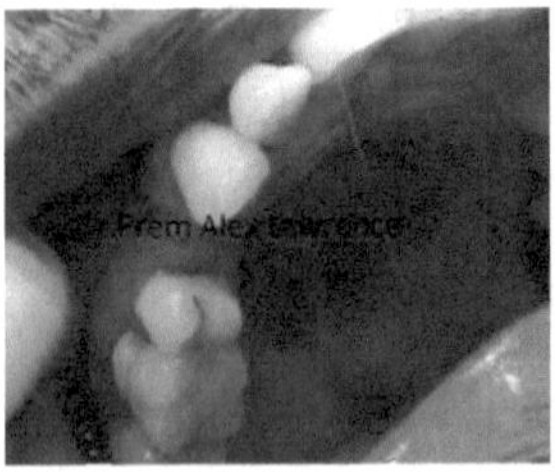

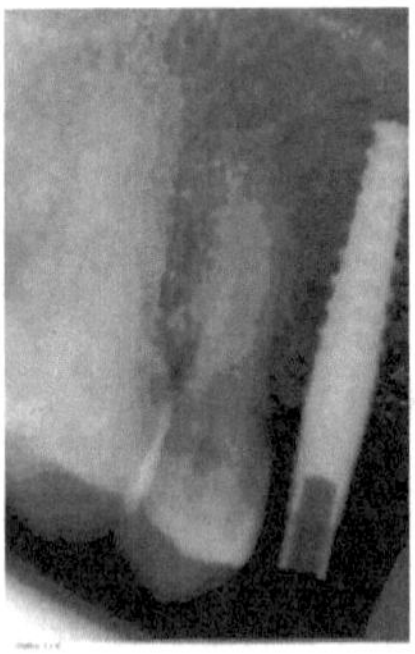

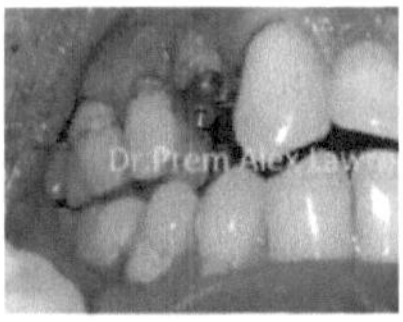

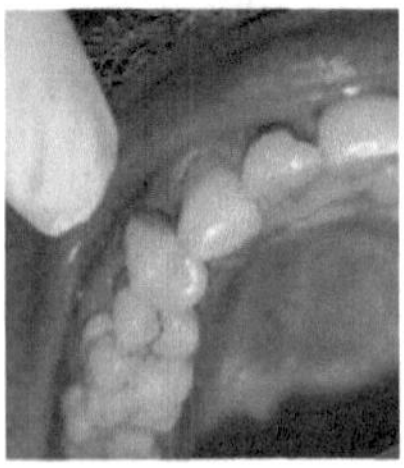

Every year, he has at least referred me to 5 patients who come searching for me and claim Gopal referred me. I have done multiple implants, crowns, and aligners on them. Briefly met him in Covid times when he got his wisdom tooth removed. Even that day, he made my surgeon wait. Habits seldom change.

But he is one of my staunch brand ambassadors who believes I am the best for him and his known people. I am blessed in that way.

Moral of The Story:

Some people don't look like diamonds themselves but make sure people around them are shining like diamonds. Selfless people, these people keep the world alive.

Be like Gopal. What goes around, comes around.

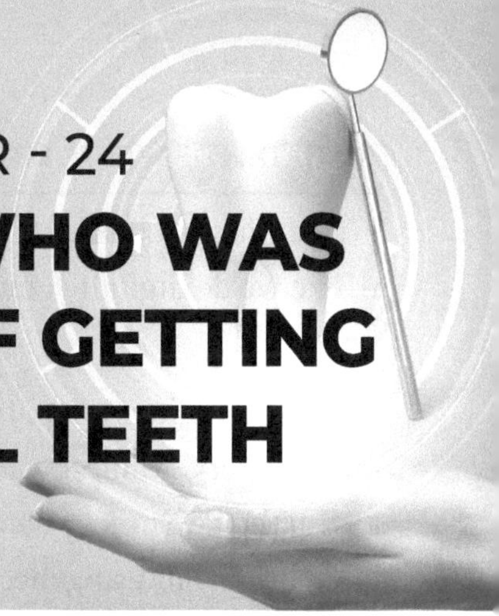

CHAPTER - 24

THE LADY WHO WAS ASHAMED OF GETTING BEAUTIFUL TEETH

Beauty is subjective. Beauty is in the eye of the beholder. Very rarely do people think being beautiful, is subject to a lot of discussion among family and friends. That is the crux of this story as well.

A 45-year-old female patient named Maheshwari* (Name Changed) came down to me from Singapore*(Country Changed) for rehabilitation of her entire mouth. She was suffering from Chronic Periodontitis (i.e. Gum Disease), and most of her teeth were shaky or with a lot of infection. This gum disease has progressed to a level where the teeth were spaced from each other, and a lot of gaps were there in her upper front teeth due to a condition called pathological migration.

Maheshwari has been living like this for more than 10 years, and she runs a retail shop. She is locally known to many, and hence, she did not want to get any treatment in her country; she wanted to get it in India.

We planned and executed the All on 4 Pro™ technique, where we do digitally guided surgery and 24-hour immediate final teeth.

I give options to patients in terms of tooth alignment after surgery. Maheshwari, too, was given what I often call a "Textbook Smile", where teeth are aligned perfectly and look bright and angelic. This will also be done with the physiologically best fit for the particular patient.

Maheshwari was thrilled at first to look at herself looking younger and with a dazzling smile. She suddenly remembered her family and friends and the people in her city. She felt if she had such a beautiful transformation, everyone would get to know her and tease her. She felt ashamed to be judged by others.

Before After

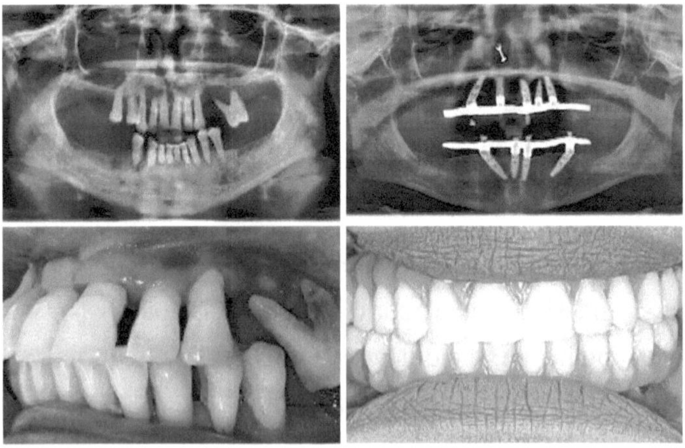

Even after my team and I had counselling her for a long, she did not want “Textbook Smile”. She wanted the teeth to align with gaps as she had previously. I gave in to her demand but told her I would do a trial.

The next day, during the trial with gapped teeth, she understood what I meant. She understood that the World would judge you however and whatever you do, and now, after all our reassurance, she was ready to take the plunge with a beautiful set of teeth without gaps.

I delivered a final Titanium frame Hybrid screw-retained prosthesis, after which one of my doctors, Dr Jananee, commented that Maheshwari looked at least 15 years younger and could be called her daughter’s elder sister now.

Maheshwari went back to her country very happy and came for a review with me during every Pongal time, and I will be meeting her this year, too.

She remains happy to date, and all her initial confusion has now turned into supreme confidence.

She smiled happily ever after.

Moral of the Story:

Many times, we live for others. We are subject to trials and judgements by everyone. But we have to live our lives and cannot live for others. People have their own yokes to handle to remember us.

With regards to smiling transformations after implants, usually, it is the family that gives the best and worst comments, and I have seen patients being misled into joy or depression due to this. It is better to ignore comments, especially after full-mouth rehabilitation.

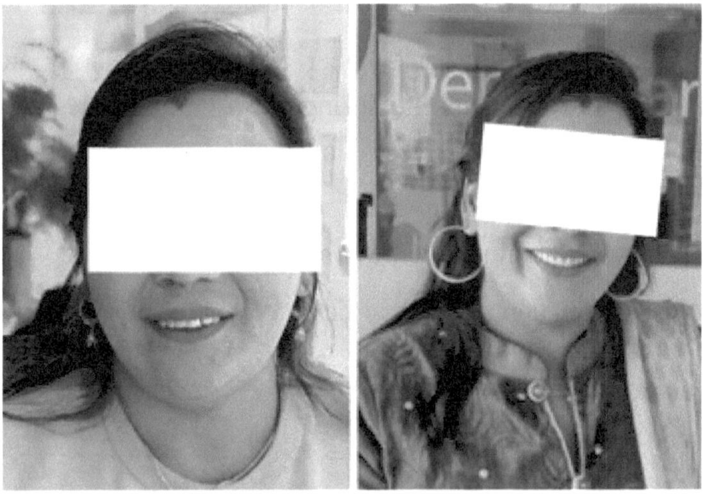

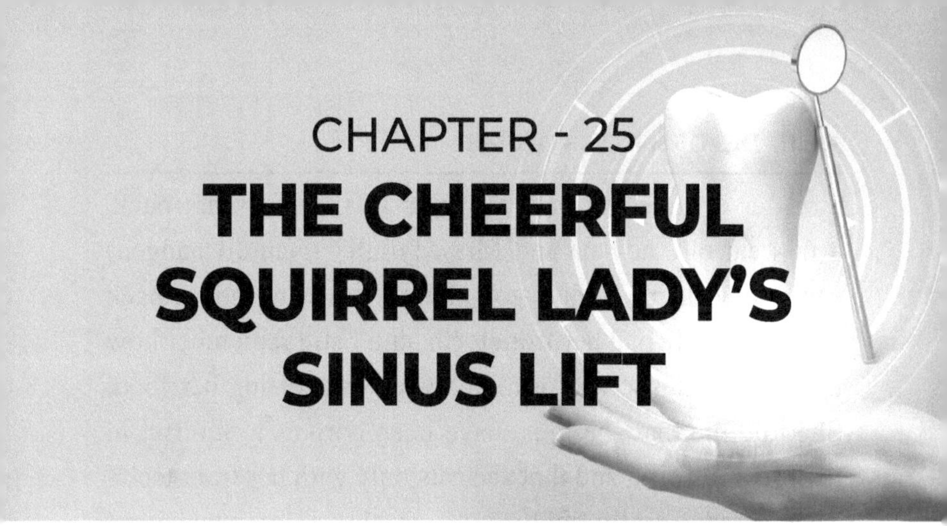

CHAPTER - 25
THE CHEERFUL SQUIRREL LADY'S SINUS LIFT

Do you know why we can walk with our heads erect even though we have thick bones in our faces and skulls? The reason is the presence of sinuses. These sinuses are just empty spaces that increase the hollowness of the bone, making it light and resulting in us being able to keep our heads erect.

Sinuses are never a friend to Implantologists. In the Indian population, they are big in the upper jaw, resulting in deficient bone for implant placement. Hence, I do a procedure termed as Sinus lift in such patients, where I access the Upper Jaw sinus directly or indirectly, push the sinus membrane up and place a lot of bone grafts. This is often associated with implant placement along the newly grafted bone, and then a crown is placed on top of the implant, usually after 5 to 6 months.

After doing thousands of Sinus lifts, three years back, a 63-year-old lady named Mrs Mythili* (Name Changed) came to visit me with a complaint of missing upper back teeth. She only had her front teeth, and I still remember how much she laughed and asked how she was eating her food. She told me that she must have been born as a Squirrel in her previous birth and that she eats only with her front teeth. That sounded really funny, and from that point, whenever I meet a patient with no back teeth, I think about this patient and Squirrels.

The thing that stood between her and her getting upper back teeth was her Upper Sinus. I planned an indirect sinus lift for her, and it was perfectly executed with a few implants in her lower jaw and a few crowns in her upper jaw. She now smiled well, ate well and practically added more fun to the already energetic person.

I recently saw her for review after 3 years, and she mentioned that she has now progressed from a Squirrel to a human. Such positive people and people who make fun of themselves keep the world going.

Moral of the Story:

Sinuses are not a bad word in Dentistry. Sinus surgeries associated with Dental Implants are very predictable.

Dont eat like a squirrel! Eat the Human Way!

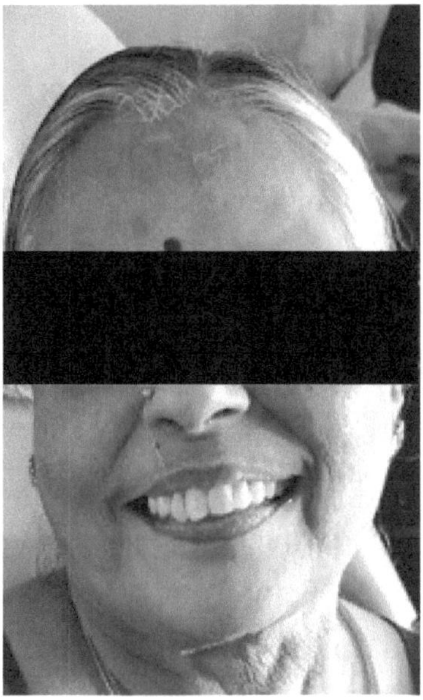

CHAPTER - 26

THE IMPLANT PLAN THAT SAVED A LIFE

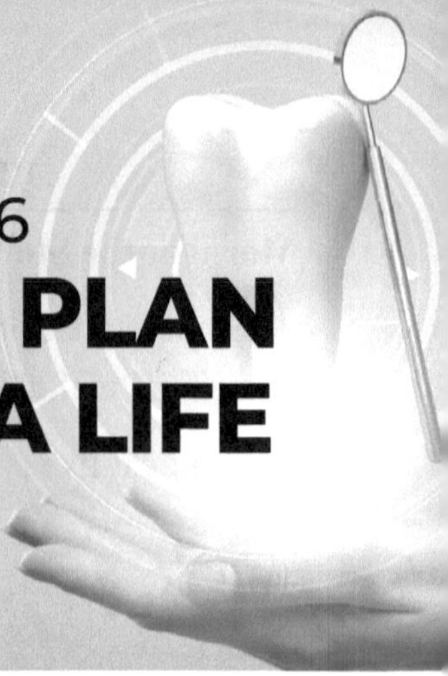

I read an article in Reader's Digest 18 years ago: " A visit to the Dentist can save your life". The article talked about how many medical issues first show signs in the Oral Cavity, aka Mouth. I have myself diagnosed hundreds of patients with underlying diabetes, which they never knew. Diabetes is known to cause Gum Diseases and usually typically presents as multiple gum abscesses.

Many diseases and infections, such as Anaemia, Lichen planus, HIV, Lupus, Pemphigus, herpes, etc, have oral manifestations and can be easily identified. The reason why a good dentist asks you to visit them at least once a year is also this.

This story involves a 55-year-old female who happens to be my close friend's mother-in-law. She had recently extracted one of her teeth elsewhere, and my friend, knowing me as an Implantologist, wanted to replace it. He also mentioned that her gums had been bleeding for some time and also wanted a consultation on that.

He brought her to my clinic, and the moment I met her and examined them, I knew something was wrong. She had patches of blood clots under her gum tissue, which was very evident, and there was spontaneous bleeding everywhere, and it didn't look like the usual gum disease. I told him to drop the Implant treatment for now and that it looked like an emergency and referred her to a known haematologist.

She was diagnosed with leukaemia, and for almost 6 months, she underwent intensive chemotherapy and recovered from the disease. I recently met my friend's wife at a birthday party, where she mentioned that her mother is alive because of me and that the Implant treatment was still pending.

Professionally, felt very happy that day!

Moral of the Story:

Yes, a routine Dental visit can save your life. The Dentist at the corner of your street can give you more insights into any medical situation you may have.

Once a year, a dentist visit can save your life...! Indeed!

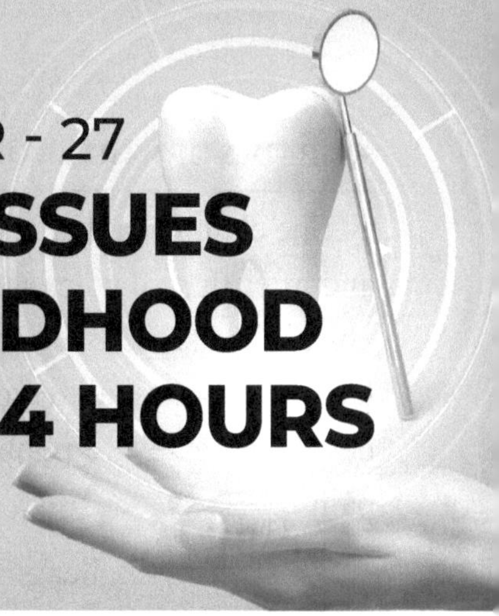

CHAPTER - 27
DENTAL ISSUES SINCE CHILDHOOD SOLVED IN 24 HOURS

Visiting a dentist as a child is crucial and exposes the child to dentists, and many future dental issues are prevented. As a kid, I remember my parents taking me to a dentist, whose clinic is on the first floor, in a place called Thingalchanthai, where I got a filling done, which very well to this day stays in my mouth. That dentist played a major role in my oral health for all these years, and I have never been scared of a dentist.

The story is similar to mine. A lady, currently 42 years old, named Kala*(Name Changed), was taken to a city college for all her dental treatments when she was a kid. Though she developed a dental phobia, her parents kept taking treatments without really analyzing them. She had undergone orthodontic braces, and recently, she claimed that without her knowledge, she was forced to undergo orthognathic surgeries (Jaw Bone is surgically cut into positions for alignment of teeth).

She claims that her brother pushed me into the treatment, and after that, she developed a lot of pain in her teeth. She always had some issue or other that warranted extraction of teeth and root canal treatments followed by crowns. She also developed a severe phobia, and she managed her life with pain.

This was a challenging case since she had also had her previous surgeries marks in bone with wires. These wires caused bone deficiency at certain points. Her left side bone was also marked with less bone. I had to avoid these wires and make use of the maximum bone available wherever.

I did an All on 4 Pro ™ concept with digital guides and 24-hour immediate teeth. I placed six implants in each arch and loaded the 4 best implants immediately since she wanted a zirconia prosthesis after 6 months.

She is now happy and getting used to her first set of teeth.

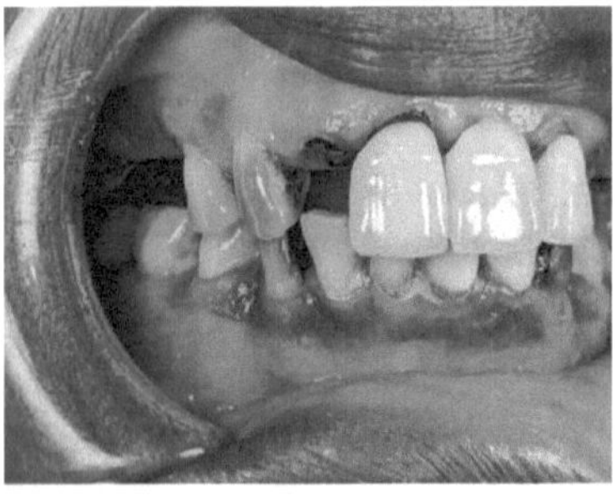

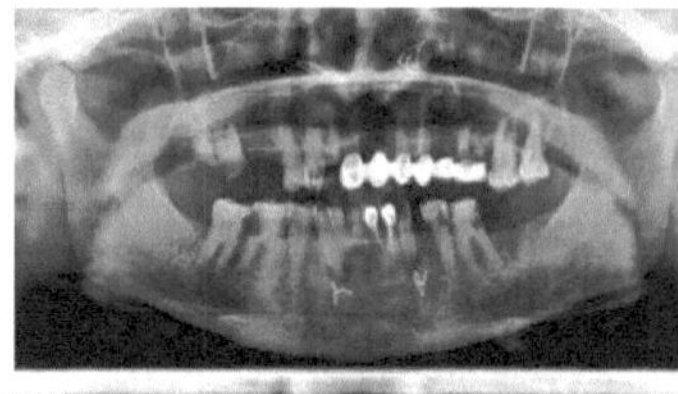

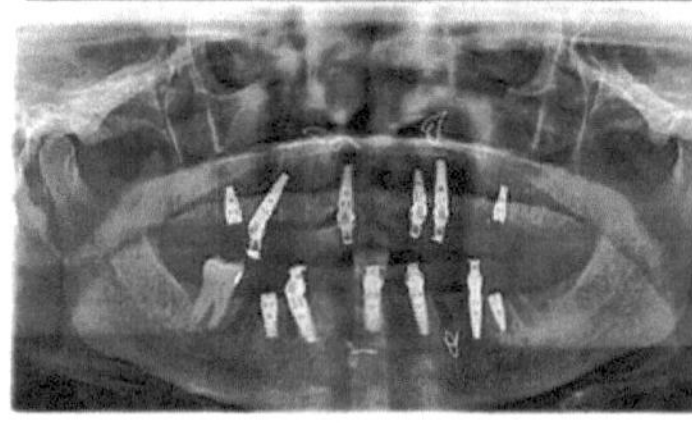

All these could have been avoided with second opinions by her family when she was a kid. I do not have her exact past dental history, but the feeling that you never know what treatment you are going to undergo, that too, a major surgery, is frightening.

Moral of the Story:

Second Opinions are not bad. Too many opinions are also bad. Second opinions give you a choice to decide on elective treatments. In this story, the patient would have probably been way better if her family had taken a second opinion.

Take second opinions! They are not a crime.

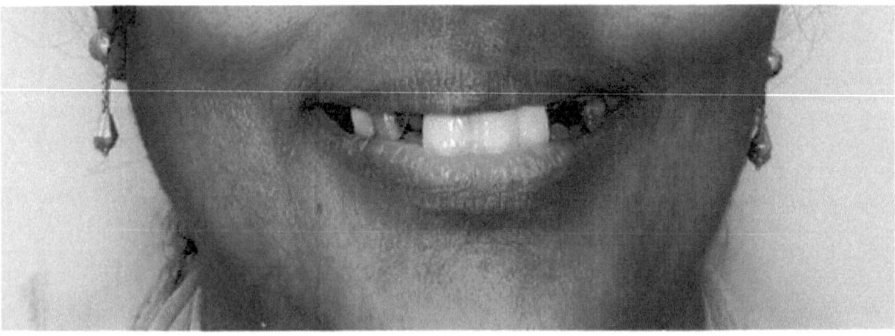

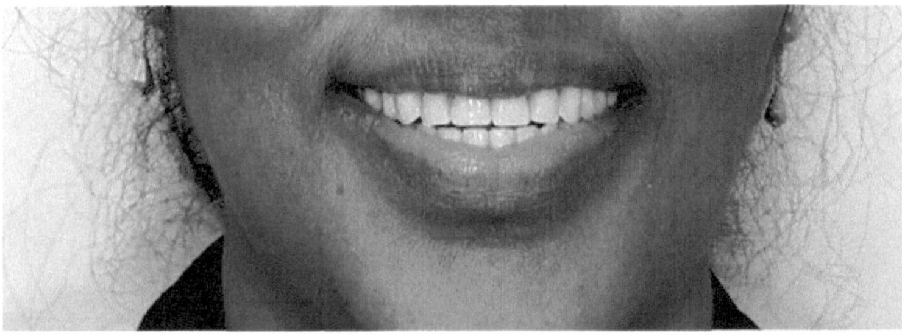

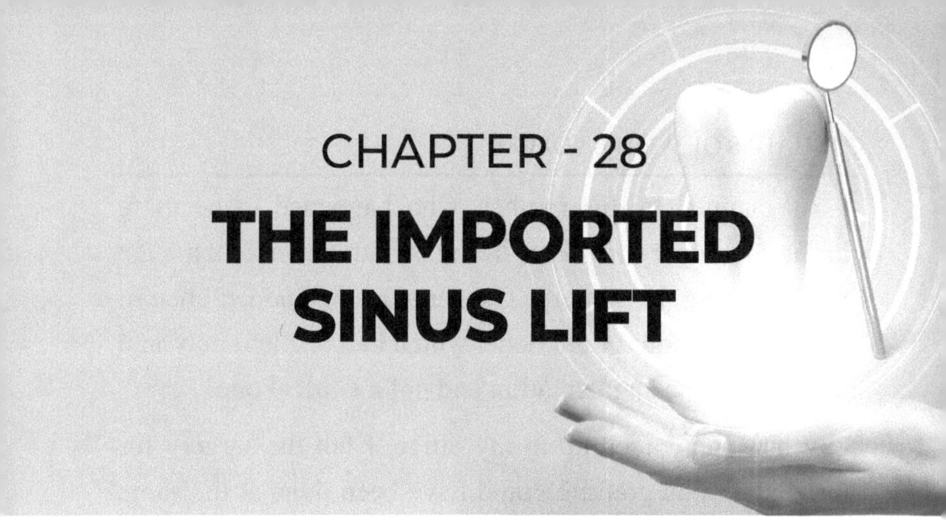

CHAPTER - 28

THE IMPORTED SINUS LIFT

Sinus Lifts are a boon to Implantologists. Whether it's around single implants, multiple implants, or zygomatic implant procedures, sinus lifts offer the best scenario for replacing teeth. I love sinus lifts, whether direct or indirect, because when in experienced hands, they are so predictable, and their outcomes are excellent.

I have a technique where very rarely I don't place an implant after a sinus lift. Inevitably, Implants are placed and grafted, and after about 6 months, the crowns are placed on sinus-lifted implants.

This is the story of a young guy named Abdul*(Name Changed) who has just completed his master's in Australia and started working there. Abdul had two of his premolars on the left side constantly in issue. They had some huge infection, and these two teeth were removed in Australia. The doctors there advised him to get implants, but alas, he did not have enough bone.

As claimed by his mother, who happened to be there during his surgery for sinus lifting, Abdul underwent a huge trauma during the surgery. The surgeons had added bone to increase the width of the bone, which had resulted only in a horizontal bone augmentation and not a vertical one.

When they ended up in my office, I felt the surgery for horizontal bone grafting could have been done at the same time to avoid two surgeries. The logic did not hit me.

I performed a sinus lift vertically, augmenting the sinus, placing implants in the sites and closing the site. Abdul's mother claimed this time, the surgery was much less traumatic, unlike his previous experience.

It healed perfectly, and I recently met Abdul after 8 months in the Christmas vacation of 2023 and could see how nicely new bone had formed and the implants taken up. I also delivered a digitally designed screw-retained crown to them.

The patient underwent two stepped surgeries, which could have been avoided had my Australian counterpart decided treatment plans were better.

Moral of the Story:

I often have felt the surgical skills and the decision-making skills of Indian doctors to be superior to our counterparts elsewhere because of the exposure and experience in several cases.

All Hail India and its medical education!

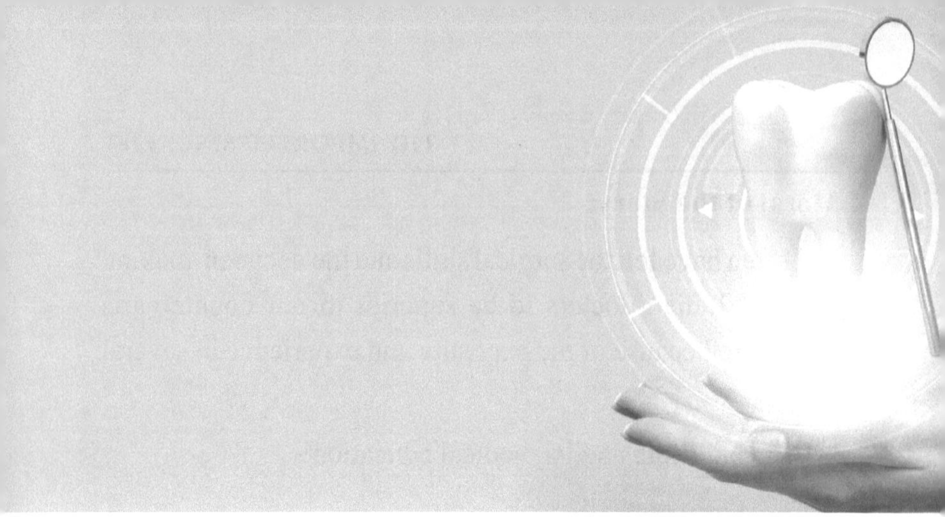

Sibling relationships are one of the best to have in life. Whenever I have been down, it has always been my brother who lifted me. There's a magical dynamic to sibling love—the playful teasing, the unspoken understanding, and the comfort found in the familiarity of shared history. It's a relationship that encompasses an entire spectrum of emotions—love, rivalry, protection, and loyalty—all intricately woven into the fabric of their connection.

I recollect two patients with whom their siblings stood rock solid during their treatments at my clinic.

One is a 43-year-old patient from Hyderabad, Ravi Reddy* (Name Changed), who had an unusual problem. He had been having shaky teeth for 15 years. The unusual problem is that his left canine tooth has been completely loose, yet he has held to it for years. That particular tooth has grown down, giving him a vampirish look, and every time he talks, it moves out and in.

I decided on full arch dental implants, and after the

decision, the sister came. The sister was very concerned about her little brother, who is 43 years old. I was amazed at the kind of care she was giving and also the way she stayed completely with the brother during the entire procedure of All on Six and Hybrid Prosthesis. Even if the patient never had any doubts, the sister came to me asking at least a few doubts every time we met.

Another sister story was of a similar-aged lady patient who came from Canada named Lavanya*(Name Changed). Lavanya had a unique issue of proclined upper front teeth, which she felt had to go and get implants done. The only issue was that she had a Dolichocephalic face (Long face), and all her front region jaw bone was so thin about 3.0mm. The smallest diameter implant I use is 3.3 mm. Hence, an immediate implant crown could not be done since the bone augmentation procedures would be required, and time was a constraint.

Before After

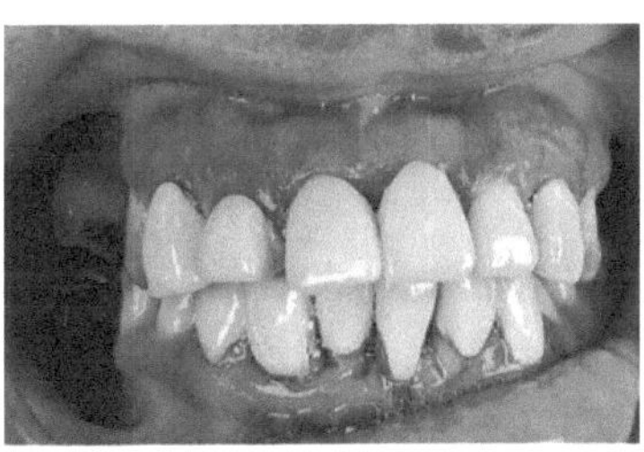

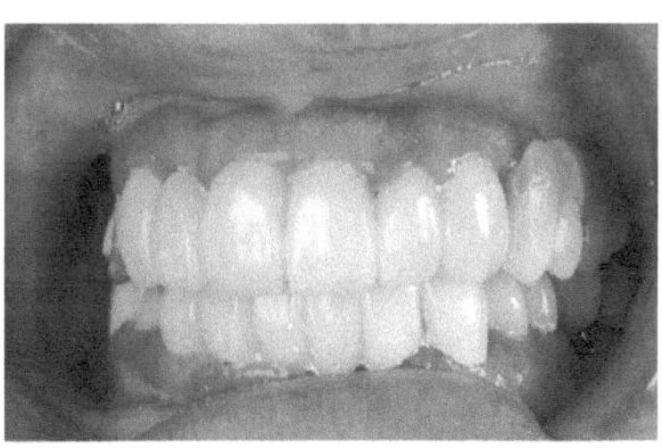

Here came the sister into play. Lavanya's sister was the one who came and told us exactly what Lavanya wanted. Lavanya wanted much straighter and more aligned teeth. The whole treatment plan changed after this. We decided on zirconia crowns in the upper front region and a combination of implants in the back region, which eventually uplifted her face, and she looked even more beautiful with regularly arranged teeth.

In these two cases, the sisters played a crucial role in the transformation of their siblings, and the care they showed throughout the procedures was heartening to see.

Moral of the Story

Sibling love weaves threads of support and understanding, stitching together moments of joy and solace. It's in the embrace of this bond that we find the strength to weather life's storms and the warmth of companionship that lights our way through the darkest of days. My own brother is a perfect example of this.

Cherish the gift of sibling love, for in its embrace lies a treasure trove of unwavering support, enduring camaraderie, and an unspoken understanding that transcends time.

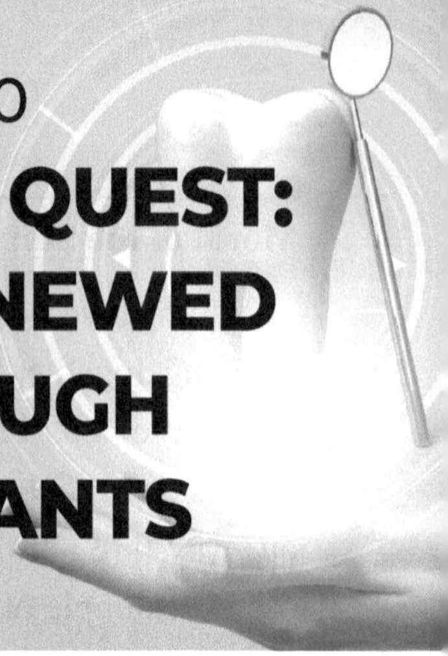

CHAPTER - 30

OCTOGENARIAN QUEST: EMBRACING RENEWED SMILES THROUGH DENTAL IMPLANTS

Amidst the ebb and flow of life, some moments stand as testaments to resilience, moments where the desire for improvement overrides the boundaries of age. In a world where technology and healthcare continue to evolve, a group of individuals emerges octogenarians, each with a singular purpose: to reclaim the joy of effortless chewing and functional comfort.

Their decision to embark on a journey toward dental implants at an age when many might consider such procedures beyond reach speaks volumes about the unwavering spirit that thrives within them. As I came to know these remarkable individuals, their stories unfolded—a tapestry of determination, wisdom, and a quest for an enhanced quality of life.

Their stories resonate with resilience, courage, and an unwavering spirit that challenges the limitations often associated with age. Join me as I unravel the narratives of these four extraordinary octogenarians (80 Years old and above), each with their unique journey towards embracing dental implants—a testament to the enduring strength of the human will and the pursuit of a better quality of life, irrespective of age.

The First Patient was 85-year-old Mr Jegadeesan*(Name Changed) with broken and decayed teeth who wanted nice teeth to chew. He told me he had broken his Fixed Deposit to get quality teeth. His daughters stood by him. He got his final teeth, and in review, he exclaimed he eats even Murukku (a Classic South Indian Snack) nowadays.

The second patient was an 83-year-old Mr Palani*(Name Changed), who retired from a Central Government Job. His request to me was that he needed good teeth to show in Video Calls to his Grandson staying in the USA. He was so satisfied that the next time his grandkids came to India, he brought them to our clinic to show all of us. Now, more than 4 years later, he still comes for yearly reviews and tells me that he almost eats everything and that he feels at least 20 years younger.

The third story is about 80-year-old Mr Krishnan*(Name Changed), who happened to read about me on a few websites and wanted to get implants done. He had broken and bad teeth and wanted to change all. He also told me all his children were now settled, and he wanted to do self-care, and that is the reason he wanted nice teeth now. Once permanent good teeth were fixed, he told me that he felt completely transformed. He now smiles and eats better.

The fourth story is about 81-year-old Mr Moorthy*(Name Changed), who also, like the previous 3 patients, decided on himself to get good teeth. He had very bad teeth that were jutting out from his mouth with shaky mobile and teeth that had huge gaps. After he got his teeth, he got his confidence back; he told me that he can eat everything and that he also pushed his daughter's father-in-law to get a similar treatment.

All the above cases had similar scenarios, and I perform similar surgeries. I do an All on Four Pro ™ technique with minimal trauma and a Hybrid prosthesis. I make sure these Hybrid Prostheses are given within a week. I keep it simple and make sure they can enjoy food as soon as possible.

These four octogenarians decided their destiny by themselves.

Moral of the Story:

Age is but a number, eclipsed by the enduring spirit that fuels our desires for a better, more fulfilling life. The decision of these octogenarians to pursue dental implants reflects the timeless truth that determination, coupled with a willingness to embrace change, knows no bounds. Their stories teach us that the pursuit of improved quality of life is a journey open to all, regardless of age, and that the quest for comfort and joy remains a fundamental aspect of the human spirit, transcending the limitations often imposed by time.

Hope we all live to see our 80s like these Gentlemen! Be like these Men!

Before *Before*

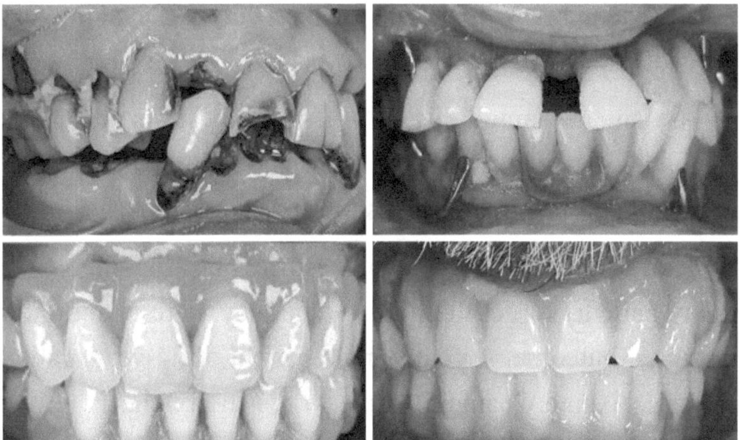

After *After*

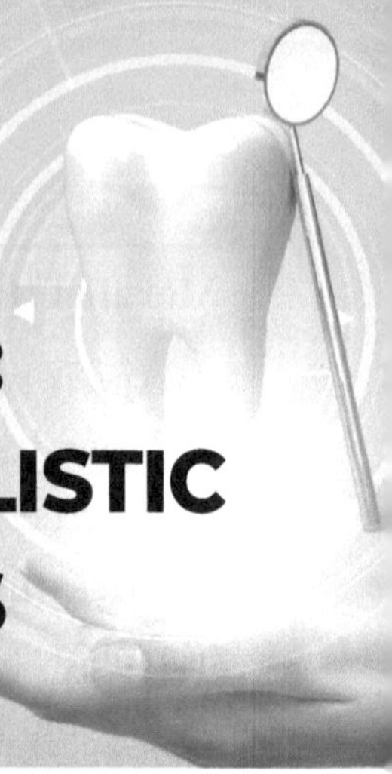

CHAPTER - 31

MANAGING EXPECTATIONS: NAVIGATING UNREALISTIC PATIENT GOALS

When people look forward to transformative dental procedures, there's a mix of hope and reality. Some patients, in their quest for a perfect smile, expect miracles that go beyond what modern dentistry can achieve. Their dreams often imagine flawless smiles and instant changes, not always in line with the practical aspects of dental implant procedures.

As an Implantologist, I've seen these expectations firsthand, observing the clash between strong hopes and the practical realities of dental restorations.

The following stories were surprising for me since many patients forget the initial stage they were in and their expected outcome. A young male patient of 24 years called Prasad* (Name Changed) came to me in crutches. He had fallen off his bike recently, and since he was not wearing a helmet, he lost his 5 front teeth in the upper jaw, and one tooth was removed to fix his broken jaw in the lower jaw. Usually, a fractured jaw and avulsed teeth would result in very thin bone and a change of shape of the bone, too.

The esthetic outcomes were explained to the patient since the bone quantity was compromised, and the bone and gum tissues had to be rebuilt. He understood everything, and I did my best to use the maximum available bone and placed implants in positions, making sure a good prosthesis could be made. Lower, too, the implant had to avoid the plates that he had to fix the broken bone.

Everything was picture perfect when suddenly, on the day of the delivery of his tooth, he turned rogue. He started whining about the bulk of the prosthesis and tooth colour and had a complaint about everything.

We sent back the crowns to the lab to adjust them to what he wanted but within physiological limits. I counselled him about that he cannot expect to transform into a model. We had to play within the limits of lost bone and reassured him that he would understand once he got used to it.

Though the prosthesis was very well made, he could not be satisfied for long. Multiple shade changes and shape changes happened during that time, and finally, we arrived at a consensus.

Prasad did not show any such attributes the day he walked in with crutches inside the clinic, but later, for some reason, his entire expectation level soared unrealistically.

Similarly, I had a full-mouth female patient aged 54 years who had high, unrealistic expectations that she wanted to transform into someone like "Nayanthara" (A famous Indian Actress) as soon as the crowns were fixed.

There was also a patient who was so particular about his trial teeth picture taken at an angle and kept comparing it with his final teeth from a different angle.

Patients tend to forget how they were initially, and the journey to reach a reasonable outcome takes a lot of work. They forget to look at the bigger picture and are mentally stuck with trivial issues.

Dont be a Prasad!

Moral of the Story:

The journey to a restored smile is a partnership built on realistic expectations and open communication. Understanding the limitations and possibilities of dental implants is crucial to achieving satisfaction and contentment. By aligning aspirations with practical outcomes, patients and practitioners forge a path toward successful dental restoration rooted in transparency, education, and mutual understanding.

CHAPTER - 32

SMILES REBORN: THE JOURNEY OF DENTAL IMPLANTS POST-JAW TUMOUR RESECTION

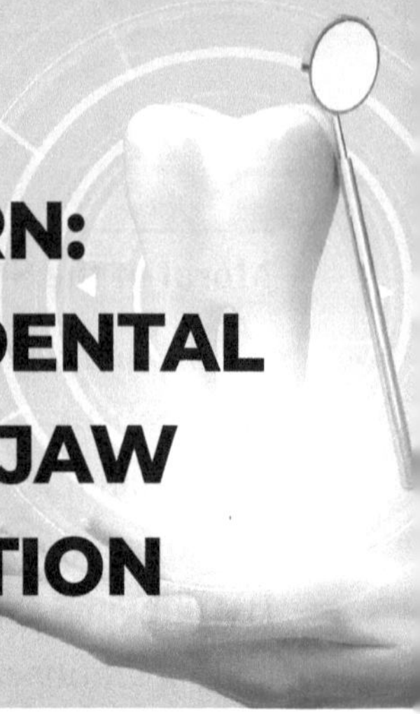

In the wake of adversity and surgical intervention for jaw tumours, a beacon of hope emerges in the form of dental implant procedures. This chapter contains two stories of individuals who, following the challenging path of tumour resection, embarked on a journey toward dental restoration. Their narratives are testaments to resilience, depicting the transformative power of dental implants in reclaiming not just smiles but a sense of normalcy and confidence.

The first story is about a little girl who is 16 years old and waiting to embark on a life journey to success. Her name is Mary*(Name Changed), and she is an aspirant to become a Chartered Accountant. She was always cheerful until tragedy struck when she was 13 years old. She was identified to have Odontogenic Keratocyst, a benign tumour in the lower jaw.

The tumour ate most of her bone, and she had to undergo a tumour resection surgery. She underwent the procedure, and after that, she had a huge defect with a few front teeth also removed. She recovered well, and after recovery, she had to attend school with no teeth. Though a temporary removable prosthesis was given, it gave only some confidence. Luckily, all her friends were very supportive.

Since there was no recurrence of the tumour in 2 years, I proceeded to place the implants in the basal bone and gave her the much-needed ceramic crowns, which were fixed, looked better and gave her all the confidence.

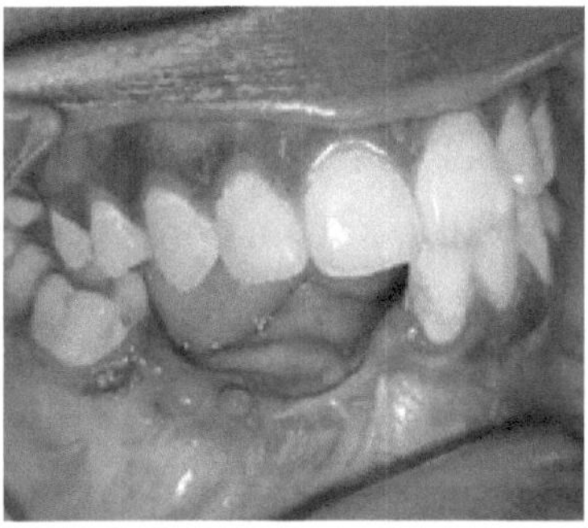

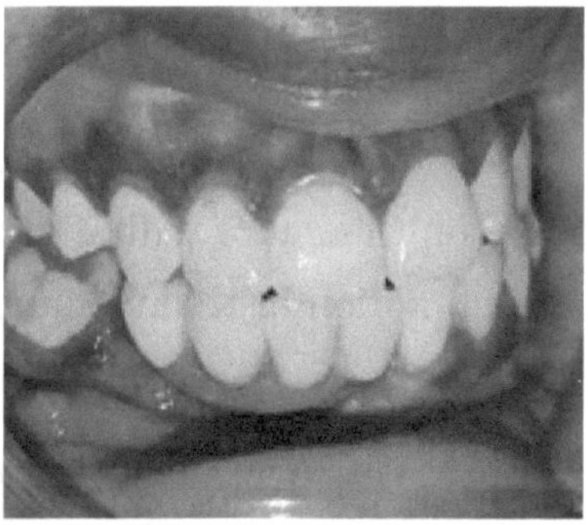

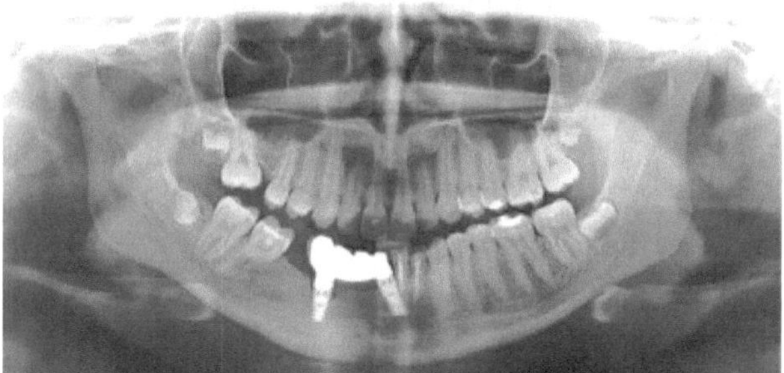

The second story is just very similar to Mary's. This was a 24-year-old Guy named Kenny*(Name Changed). Kenny also had a similar Odontogenic Keratocyst 2 years back and had been operated on. Kenny, when he came to me, had very little bone and was suggested by a different hospital to undergo implants in a two-step process of bone grafting and later implants. Kenny's mom was worried since they were on the lookout for a bride for him, and they did not want to wait for one year.

When they came to me, I explained both the techniques of grafting and waiting or doing implants with the compromised bone but will have to be watchful over the years. They took the second route, where I placed Nobel Active ® Implants and went on to restore with a great-looking zirconia prosthesis. Within a month, Kenny came to meet me with his wedding invite.

Both cases posed technical difficulties, yet the implant and surgical skills and the patience of these patients resulted in a wonderful outcome.

Moral of the Story

The human spirit, indomitable in the face of adversity, finds solace and renewal through the transformative power of dental implants. These stories reflect the resilience within us, showcasing that even after the challenges of jaw tumour surgeries, the path to restored smiles and regained confidence exists. They stand as reminders of the unwavering determination and hope that pave the way for a brighter, more fulfilling life, illustrating that even amidst hardship, the possibility of renewal and restoration shines through.

Be like Mary and Kenny in Tough Times!

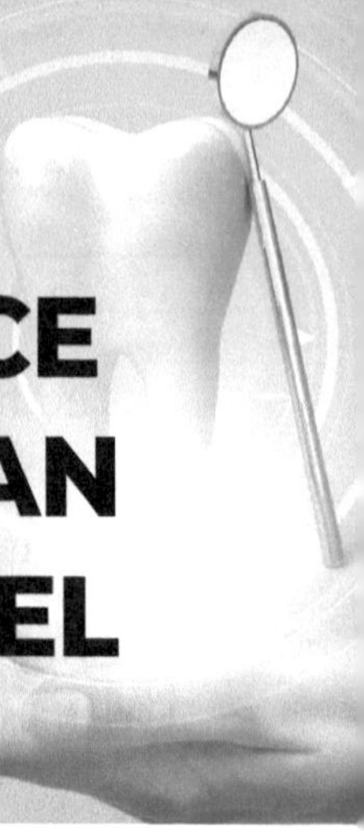

CHAPTER - 33

A SECOND CHANCE AT 31 YEARS FOR AN ARMED PERSONNEL

In the labyrinth of life's unexpected turns, Veera* (Name Changed) found himself grappling with a dental dilemma at the tender age of 31. This is the poignant tale of a young man who lost more than just teeth, only to discover a remarkable second chance through the transformative power of dental implants. Join us as we unravel the threads of Veera's journey, exploring the emotional valleys and triumphant peaks that accompany the restoration of a smile and a life.

Veera serves in the Indian Army. He was posted in the borders, and from the borders, we received a call asking for implants since his teeth were becoming shaky over time. We fixed an appointment to meet during his vacation, and as soon as he got back from his vacation, he landed in Chennai to meet me.

It was a classic case of aggressive Periodontitis (Gum Disease) where most of his lower jaw teeth were infected, and his upper front teeth were badly infected with severe pus draining from them. I decided to preserve a few of his upper teeth owing to his age. I also told him to be vigilant and be prepared for the failure of the remaining teeth, which may warrant implants later.

The surgery went smoothly and gave him his upper zirconia Malo Bridges, which made him look and smile better. Lower, I gave him crowns, which improved his aesthetics as well as his confidence.

He left for his work from vacation happy and better.

Losing teeth so early in life puts people in tatters. This man likes fighting for the country, and he also took steps to fight his dental issues and get them better.

Moral of the Story:

In the kaleidoscope of life's challenges, Veera's journey reminds us that resilience and courage can emerge even from the seemingly mundane corners of our existence. Through the lens of dental adversity, this chapter imparts a powerful lesson. Veera's story encourages us to face life's unexpected turns with grace, embracing the opportunities for growth and self-discovery that often accompany even the most daunting challenges.

Be like Veera!

Before

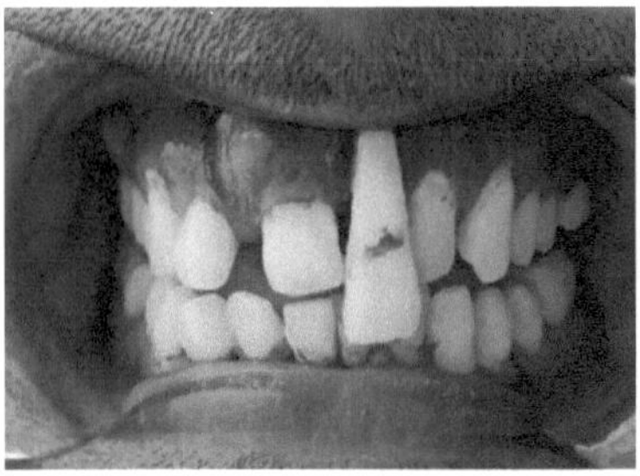

After

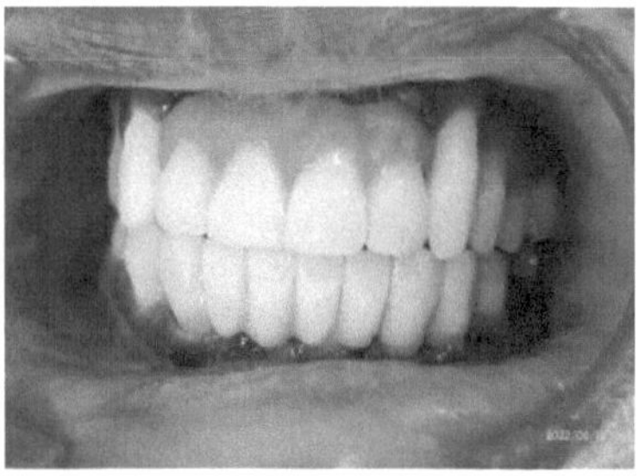

CHAPTER - 34

RECLAIMING YOUTHFUL SMILES: RESTORATION AFTER DENTAL NEGLECT

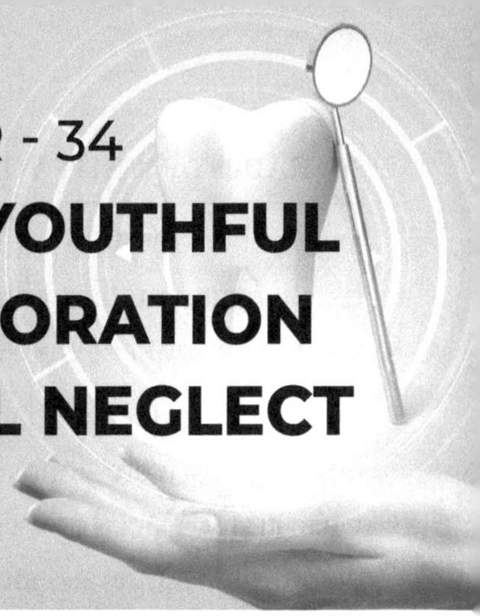

In the pursuit of youth's carefree pleasures, some inadvertently neglect the guardians of their smiles. This chapter unveils the poignant story of a young individual who, in the whirlwind of youthful abandon, unintentionally subjected their dentition to neglect and mistreatment. Amidst regrets and a desire for redemption, this individual embarks on a heartfelt journey toward dental restoration. Join me as we explore this narrative, a testament to the power of resilience and the pursuit of rectifying past neglect, paving the way for a renewed and vibrant smile.

Vivek*(Name Changed), a 24-year-old Software Professional, came to me with a unique problem. He had good teeth as a child, but all the abuse started with chocolates, as claimed by him, and improper oral health measures. He started developing multitudes of decays, a few of which his father got removed as a young kid.

The rest had a problem. He had good smiling teeth, but the posterior or back teeth were either missing or decayed and broken. He told me that he was feeling extremely old, like his grandmother, since his diet included only soft foods, and he was not able to eat any sort of hard foods.

On clinical examination, it was a collapsed bite. The upper gums were almost hitting the lower gums, and there wasn't any space for a crown to be placed. Hence, I had to do multiple surgeries, including reshaping the bone to create space, sinus lifts and bone grafting alongside.

I executed what I had planned for him and then proceeded to place crowns in the implants after 6 months. Vivek could now have the comfort of biting a few harder foods since childhood. The story also reinforced the faith in the current generation that they also want to take care of their health once they start earning. Though the abuse was in childhood, the future looks bright.

Moral of the Story

Neglect may shadow youth's carefree moments, but the pursuit of restoration shines a light of redemption. Mistakes of the past pave the way for a commitment to dental care, fostering a brighter, healthier smile. Through diligence and rectification, even neglected dentition finds its chance for renewal and rejuvenation.

Be like Vivek!

Before

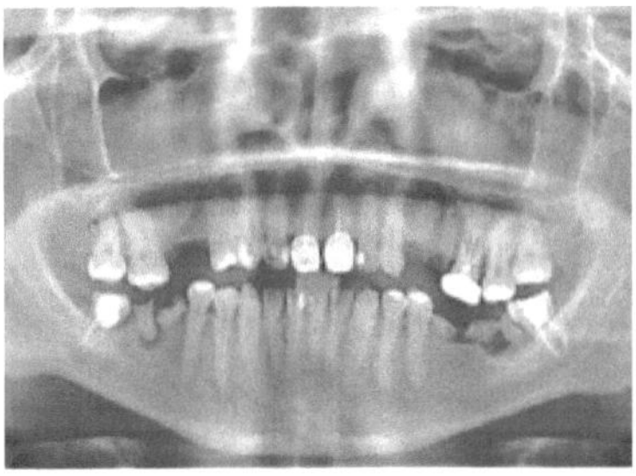

After

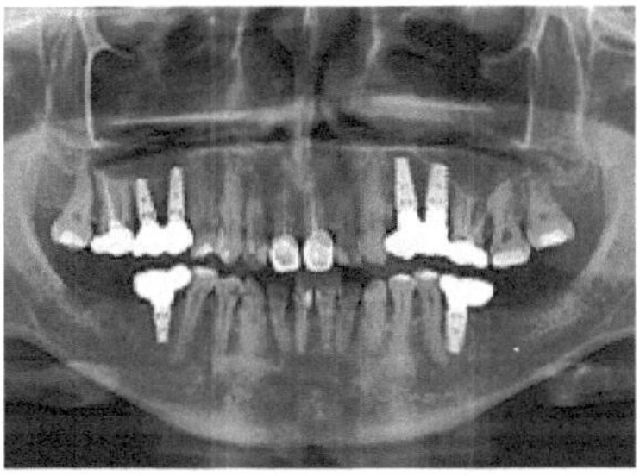

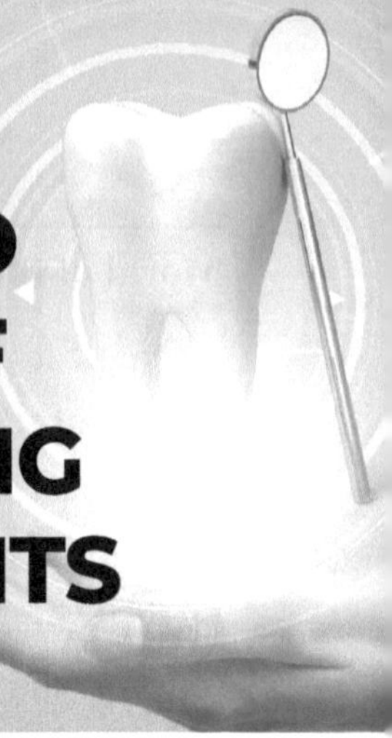

CHAPTER - 35
THE GUY WHO GOT LAID OFF BEFORE GETTING DENTAL IMPLANTS

In the ebb and flow of life, sometimes our struggles present themselves in unexpected forms. Meet Jason* (Name Changed), a resilient soul who faced the dual challenge of unemployment and dental woes. Just as the weight of job loss threatened to crush his spirit, a silver lining emerged, leading Jason on a journey from professional setback to a radiant, restored smile. This chapter unravels the narrative of perseverance, reinvention, and the transformative power of dental implants.:

Jason, a 35-year-old software professional, visited me to get his dental checkup done. He was referred by a friend, and since Jason was to be sent abroad for a project in his company the next month. He had a couple of missing back teeth and a few root canals to be done. I had planned the implant surgery the following week.

Unfortunately, he found himself at an unexpected crossroads when the company he had dedicated a decade to suddenly downsized the very next day after our implant treatment planning. Unemployment struck with a force that reverberated not only through his career but also through his personal life. As he grappled with the harsh realities of job hunting, an equally daunting challenge surfaced – his deteriorating dental health.

Unable to secure dental implants during his employment crisis, Jason navigated interviews and networking events with a diminished sense of self-confidence. Yet, with resilience as his guide, he secured a new position within three months. The first pay check marked not only a professional comeback but also the opportunity to address the dental concerns that had lingered during the job hunt.

This chapter delves into the emotional turbulence of unemployment, the impact on self-esteem, and the intricate decisions involved in prioritizing dental health amid financial uncertainties. Jason's story unfolds as he takes the reins of his life, deciding that the first investment post-employment turmoil would be in his smile.

He visited me, got his implants and crowns in 4 months, and during his recent visit for review, he did tell me he was going to Canada for a Project, and he may not return for the next 3 years. I was really happy that life came full circle, and Jason was extremely pleased as he fought his way up.

Moral of the Story

Jason's journey serves as a testament to the indomitable spirit that can emerge even in the face of simultaneous professional and personal challenges. His story teaches us that setbacks are not roadblocks but opportunities for reinvention. By choosing to invest in his dental health amidst financial uncertainties, Jason discovered that sometimes, the first step towards a brighter future begins with a confident smile. This story invites readers to embrace resilience, prioritize self-care, and recognize that even in the darkest moments, there is potential for profound transformation.

Be like Jason.

CHAPTER - 36

BEYOND THE BADGE - A POLICE CONSTABLE'S SMILE OF RESILIENCE

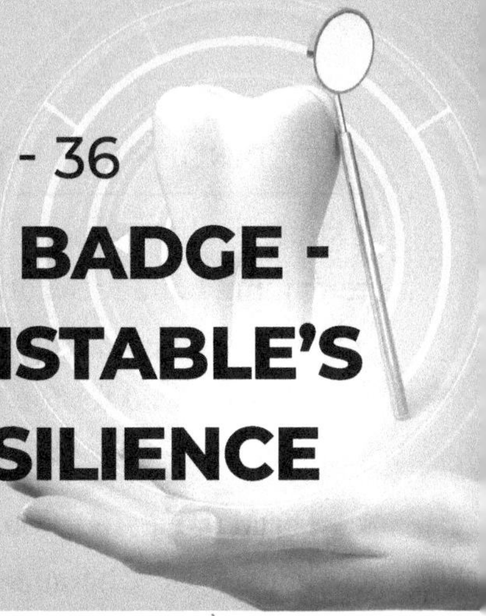

In the bustling world of law enforcement, where stoicism is often a shield, emerges the story of Cheran* (Name Changed), a police constable whose silent battle with severe gum disease threatened not only his oral health but also his confidence. This chapter unfolds the journey of a humble and reserved officer, showcasing the unexpected challenges he faced, the innovative dental solution that restored his smile, and the resilience that defines the men and women who wear the badge.

Cheran, a dedicated police constable, bore the weight of his duty with unwavering strength. However, behind the badge, he silently battled a formidable adversary – severe gum disease that had ravaged the lower left side of his jaw, leading to significant bone loss. The prospect of traditional implant placement, with compromised aesthetics, loomed as the only solution.

In a unique twist, I opted for an unconventional approach. Recognising the challenge of extensive bone loss,

I strategically extracted a semi-infected tooth, utilising the remaining bone to secure an implant at an optimal position. The innovative treatment not only addressed the gum disease but also allowed for the placement of zirconia teeth over the implants, restoring Cheran's smile almost immediately.

Throughout the journey, I gained insights into the challenges of Cheran's profession. VIP duties and Non-stop 60-hour shifts were not uncommon, often causing him to reschedule appointments. His dedication to his duty paralleled his commitment to restoring his smile, creating a narrative that transcends the dental chair into the demanding world of law enforcement.

Moral of the Story

Cheran's story illuminates the resilience that defines those who serve in law enforcement. His silent struggle with gum disease and the demanding nature of his job underscores the importance of understanding and addressing the unique challenges faced by individuals in high-stress professions. Beyond dentistry, Cheran's narrative serves as a tribute to the unsung heroes in uniform, highlighting their silent battles and the power of a confident smile in facing life's challenges.

Salute to Cheran.

Before

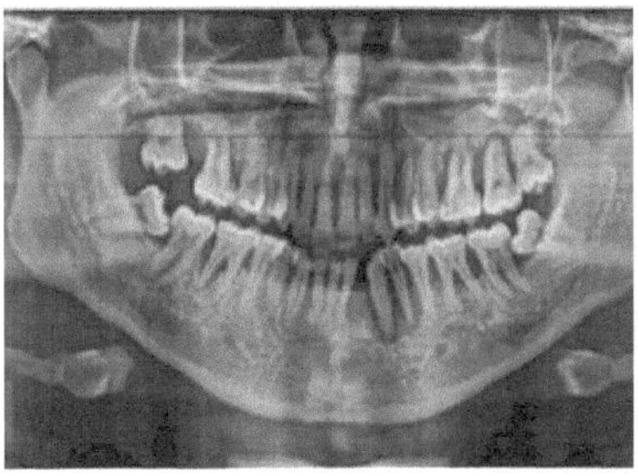

After

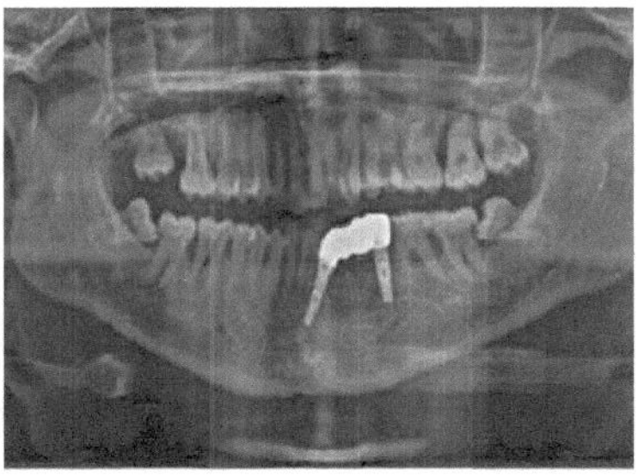

CHAPTER - 37

BRIDGING CONFIDENCE - PATIENT'S EVOLUTION FROM DOUBT TO TRUST

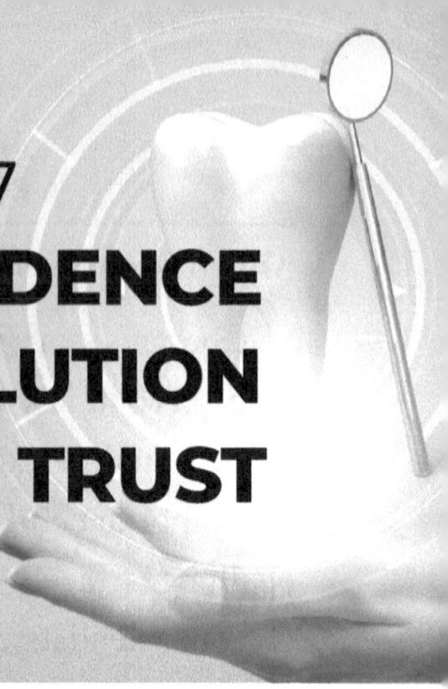

Five years ago, Anand*(Name Changed) walked into my dental clinic with a simple decay issue, armed with a surprising request – he wanted the tooth extracted and replaced with an implant. Recognising the importance of preserving natural teeth, I opted for conservative treatment, providing him with excellent composite tooth restorations instead. Little did I know that this seemingly routine decision would become the foundation for a transformative journey.

Over the years, Anand has faced another dental issue unrelated to our initial encounter. This time, he approached me with a newfound trust, convinced that an implant was the solution. The change in his perspective was remarkable – a testament to the impact of our earlier conservative approach. The small treatment plan that prioritised his natural teeth had earned him confidence.

I placed two implants in his lower arch and proceeded to give screw-retained crowns in them. The implants relieved him of the constant pain that he had over years in these teeth, which were root canal treated and crowned previously.

As we embarked on the implant procedure, Anand's trust in my expertise extended beyond dental matters. He began seeking advice on business decisions, recognising a broader sense of trust beyond the dental chair. The journey from scepticism to confidence unfolded not only in the dental clinic but also in our evolving professional relationship.

Moral of the Story

Anand's story teaches us that the foundation of trust is often built on seemingly small decisions. Prioritising conservative dental treatments not only preserved Anand's natural teeth but laid the groundwork for a strong patient-dentist relationship. Beyond the realm of dentistry, Anand's transition from a sceptical dental patient to seeking business advice underlines the broader impact of trust in professional relationships. It emphasises the idea that a foundation of trust can extend beyond the specific expertise of a professional, fostering a connection that goes beyond the surface.

Happy Patient and Happy Doctor.

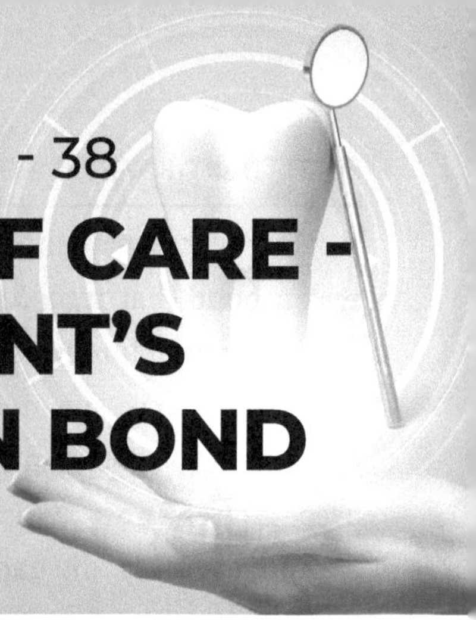

CHAPTER - 38
THREADS OF CARE - A PATIENT'S UNSPOKEN BOND

In the heart of our implant practice, amidst the hum of drills and the scent of sterilisers, an unexpected bond blossomed with a remarkable patient – Mrs. Lakshmi Gupta*(Name Changed). A 60-year-old soul with terminal dentition in her upper jaw, her journey unfolded into a unique tale of attachment and companionship. This chapter delves into the profound impact of dental implants on Mrs. Gupta's life, the surprising threads of affection that wove through her interactions with the clinic team, and the delicate balance of professionalism and personal connection.

Mrs. Lakshmi Gupta arrived at our clinic with a dental condition that demanded an extensive intervention. Terminal dentition in her upper jaw necessitated the placement of All Four implants, accompanied by a Hybrid Prosthesis, offering her a new lease on dental health. Simultaneously, her lower front teeth, plagued by gum disease, were replaced with two implants and a zirconia bridge.

However, what unfolded after the successful treatment was a bond that transcended the dental chair. Mrs. Gupta, grappling with loneliness, found solace in our clinic. Despite our admonitions, she ingeniously discovered reasons to visit, bringing bags laden with gifts – fruits, chocolates, books, and assorted treasures – expressions of gratitude and, perhaps, an attempt to bridge the gap of solitude in her life.

Understanding her need for companionship, our team welcomed Mrs. Gupta's visits, acknowledging that sometimes, healthcare extends beyond clinical procedures. The awkwardness of the situation faded into the warmth of shared moments, and gradually, our clinic became not just a place of dental care but a sanctuary of human connection for Mrs. Gupta.

Moral of the Story

Mrs. Lakshmi Gupta's story sheds light on the often-overlooked aspect of geriatric patient care – the need for human connection. Her attachment to the clinic and the team wasn't just about dental implants; it was a lifeline to combat loneliness. The chapter encourages healthcare professionals to recognise the emotional needs of patients, especially in the geriatric demographic, and to approach care with empathy and understanding.

While the exchange of gifts may seem awkward in a clinical setting, it serves as a poignant reminder that, beyond the confines of diagnosis and treatment, patients seek a sense of belonging. Mrs Gupta's tale is a testament to the transformative power of genuine human connection in the realm of healthcare.

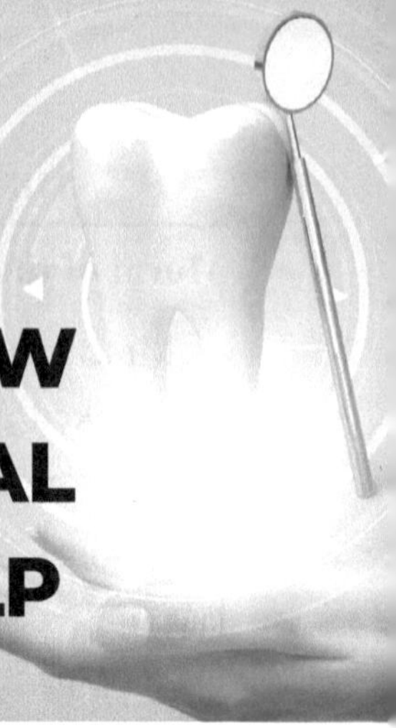

CHAPTER - 39

RESILIENCE IN SIMPLICITY - HOW REGULAR DENTAL CHECK-UPS HELP

Meet Anbu, a 50-year-old man whose journey through dental challenges paints a portrait of humility, resilience, and unwavering commitment to his oral health. Eight years ago, he became my patient when I placed an implant to replace his upper premolar. Anbu, a man of few words with a stutter in his speech, emerged as a diligent attendee of his annual dental reviews.

Two years back, our routine check-up unearthed a more complex issue – an infected central incisor with bone involvement and root resorption. Anbu's unique challenge demanded an unconventional surgical approach. With meticulous precision, I preserved the remaining gum architecture and initiated a bone surgery, creating a window above the tooth for access. The infected area was cleaned, and a delicate dance of bone grafts, membrane placement, and immediate implantation unfolded, crowned immediately with a temporary tooth. Four months later, a permanent zirconia tooth adorned Anbu's radiant smile.

Anbu's response to the treatment was not just one of physical healing but a testament to the resilience that simplicity and humility can foster. His commitment to regular reviews and his newfound confidence transformed him into a living testament to the power of meticulous dental care.

Moral of the Story

Anbu's journey underscores the significance of individualised, meticulous care in dental practice. The unconventional surgical approach became a bridge to his restored natural smile, proving that resilience often lies in simplicity. Beyond the technical success of the surgery, Anbu's commitment to his oral health, despite personal challenges, serves as an inspiration.

Be like Anbu

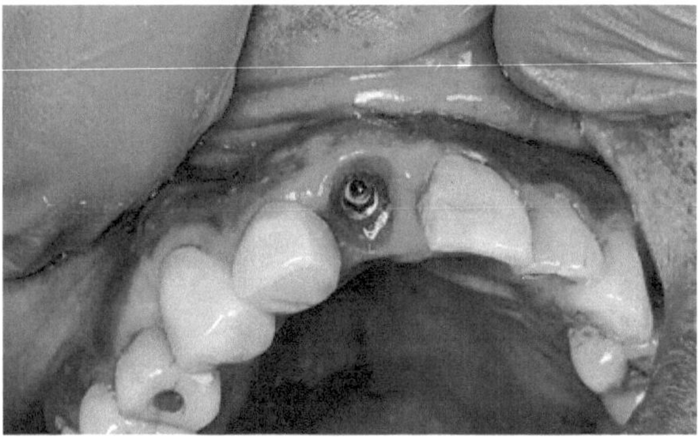

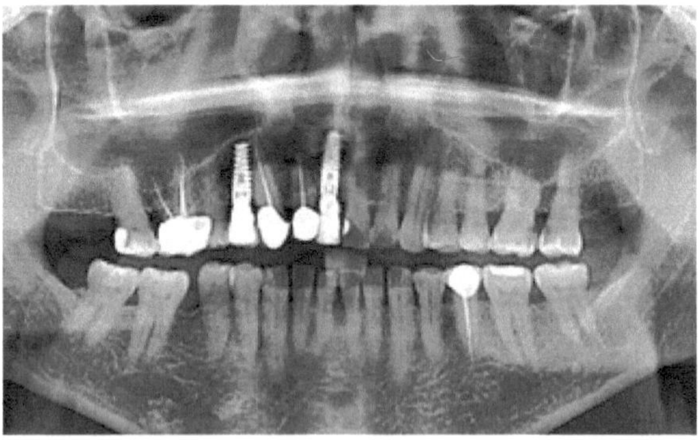

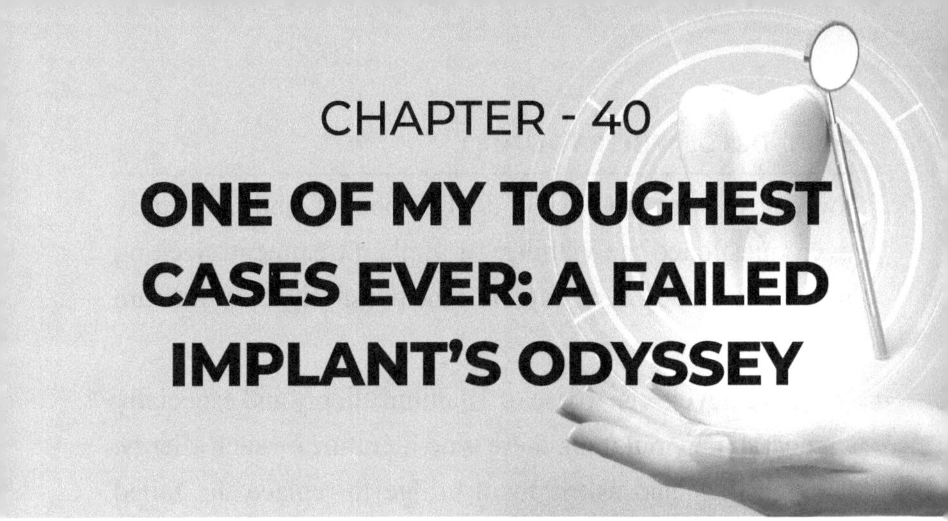

CHAPTER - 40

ONE OF MY TOUGHEST CASES EVER: A FAILED IMPLANT'S ODYSSEY

This tale of Aishwarya* (Name Changed), a 22-year-old girl, stands as a testament to her resilience and undying spirit. Six years ago, Aishwarya came to us with an infected front tooth, which had been removed. Simultaneously, she was undergoing orthodontic treatment to address minor alignment issues. Upon the completion of orthodontics, we embarked on what seemed to be a routine implant procedure.

The initial implant surgery was seemingly perfect, and in three months, Aishwarya adorned a new crown that harmonised flawlessly with her smile. However, to our collective dismay, after six months, the implant failed. As a practitioner dedicated to perfection, the failure posed a challenge that tested both my clinical skills and unwavering determination.

Undeterred by the setback, I saw an opportunity to turn adversity into triumph. Grafting the site, we patiently waited for six months before making a second attempt. Aishwarya's journey was far from easy; doubts loomed, and her family even questioned the viability of implant treatment. Seeking reassurance, they even explored the possibility of a titanium allergy.

I have never seen a case of Titanium allergy and especially in the Indian population, there is no literature on such allergy. Though they had asked for a bridge to replace the failed implant, I stood my ground to redo the implant procedure.

However, amidst the scepticism, Aishwarya and her family chose to place their trust in my expertise. The second implant procedure unfolded, and today, Aishwarya not only enjoys a problem-free implant but also flaunts a crown that complements her radiant smile.

Moral of the story:

Aishwarya's narrative echoes the trauma and challenges she faced on her journey to a perfect smile. It illuminates the psychological toll that dental setbacks can have on a patient, emphasising the importance of empathy and understanding in dental care. The ability to turn setbacks into opportunities for improvement, coupled with the trust and collaboration between patient and practitioner, serves as a profound lesson.

In dentistry, as in life, setbacks are not the end but rather a path to growth and achievement. Aishwarya's story serves as a reminder for me to remain humble no matter how high we may soar.

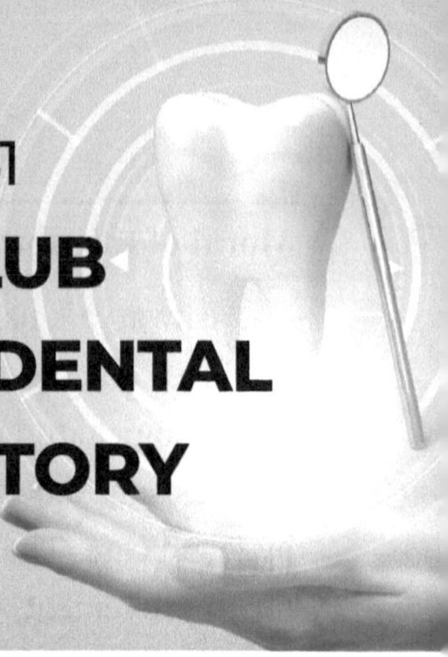

CHAPTER - 41

A ROTARY CLUB CONNECTION - A DENTAL REDEMPTION STORY

In the vibrant realm of the Rotary Club, where bonds of service and friendship intertwine, Vasan* (Name Changed), a 43-year-old member, found himself facing an unexpected dental predicament. A trusted fellow Rotarian, also a dentist, undertook the responsibility of addressing Vasan's dental issue in the front tooth. Little did Vasan know that this seemingly routine procedure would set the stage for a journey marked by challenges, redemption, and an unexpected Rotary connection.

Within 10 days of the initial dental intervention, Vasan found himself grappling with pain and a disconcerting swelling. Seeking a solution, he turned to the vast landscape of the internet, where fate led him to my clinic. Upon examination, it became apparent that the implant, placed by his fellow Rotarian dentist, was not ideally positioned. It was shorter than optimal and slightly outside the bone, rendering it susceptible to infection and preventing proper integration.

Understanding the critical nature of the situation, I

proposed a comprehensive solution – the removal of the ill-fitted implant and the placement of a longer, more suitable one. The challenge arose from the fact that the previous dentist had used the only stock of implants available, which was insufficient for an anterior implant immediately after tooth extraction. In my clinic, where a diverse range of implants in all sizes is readily available, the ideal treatment plan could be executed seamlessly.

After cleaning and grafting the site, a longer implant found its place, promising not only functional restoration but also an aesthetically pleasing result. Vasan, once embarrassed by the turn of events, learned that I shared a common bond with him as a fellow Rotarian and a Past President of a prestigious club. The shared affiliation helped alleviate any lingering discomfort, and Vasan's journey toward dental redemption took a positive turn.

Moral of the story:

Vasan's story brings to light the delicate balance between professional relationships and the pursuit of optimal patient care. The narrative underscores the importance of having a diverse inventory of resources at hand to address varying patient needs promptly. Also, Choose an Implantologist who is ever ready!

Before

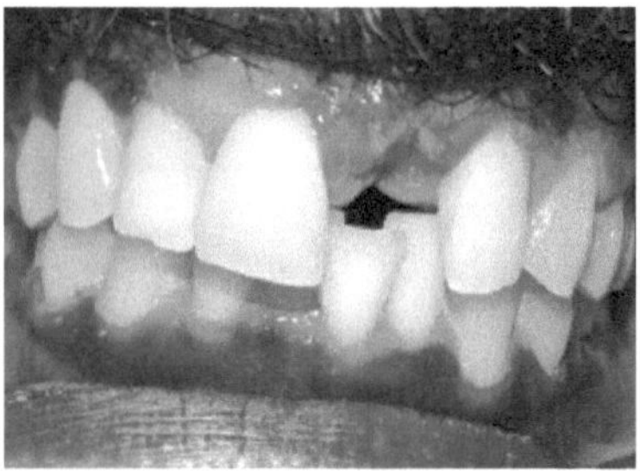

After

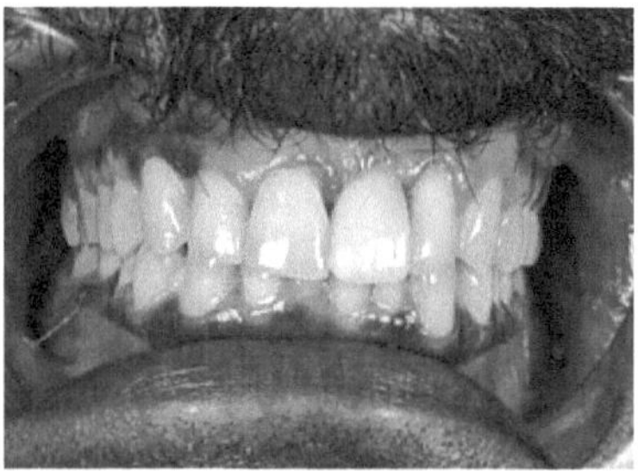

CHAPTER - 42

ONE PATIENT TO WHOM I LOST MY COOL

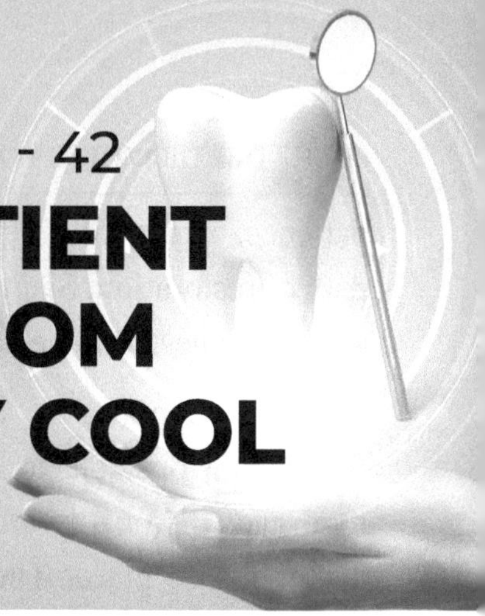

Life often throws unexpected challenges our way, testing the limits of our resilience. Enter Kumari* (Name Changed), a 32-year-old mother whose life took an unforeseen turn in a bike accident that left her and her two children with more than just physical scars. Kumari's story is one of initial reluctance, anxiety, and a daunting bone defect that seemed insurmountable.

Kumari, a meticulous and anxious individual, found herself in the throes of uncertainty after a bike accident that robbed her of her front tooth, leaving a void not just in her smile but in her confidence. Two of her children also bore the brunt of the accident, compounding the emotional toll on the family. And all this happened because neither she nor her children wore helmets.

As an Implantologist, I encountered a unique challenge with Kumari – her initial reluctance to consider dental implants. Overwhelmed by anxiety, she struggled to absorb the advice and options presented to her. It took time, patience, and gentle persuasion to guide her towards the path of restoration. She was so negative and did not take any advice suggested to her.

Upon examination, a significant bone defect posed a formidable obstacle to the implant process. Her adjacent tooth was also badly affected, which she had gotten wired in her native place. Though I advised her to get that too removed, she did not agree. She had her own treatment plan. I never lost my cool with patients, but when she did not understand the extent of her problem, I lost it. I told her since it was elective treatment, she had all rights to reject any treatment and the choice to get treatment anywhere.

I never expected, though, that she would turn around. I was pretty surprised that she had called and fixed an appointment with me the following week. I told her the treatment would follow my plan and not hers, yet I did not touch the adjacent tooth, yet I educated her that it was failing as well.

Kumari's case required extensive bone grafts and membrane placement to create a suitable foundation for the implants. Despite her initial apprehensions, Kumari surprised everyone by committing to the treatment plan. Now, as we enter the waiting period before crowning the implant, Kumari's story becomes a testament to the importance of wearing helmets.

On the last visit, when we were talking about helmets, she still told me that she would not wear a helmet in the future and was willing to risk it all. I had no words.

Moral of the story:

The only moral here is that road accidents change people's lives overnight. Wear helmets and Seat belts. Take care of your children. Never lose your cool like me.

Don't be a Kumari!

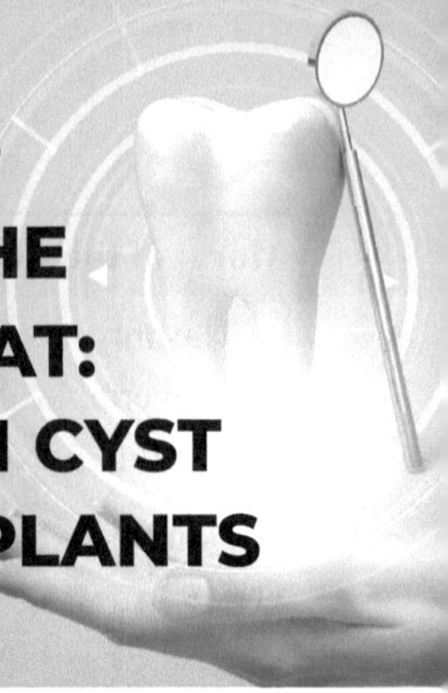

CHAPTER - 43

UNVEILING THE HIDDEN THREAT: A JOURNEY FROM CYST DISCOVERY TO IMPLANTS

In the bustling routine of a dental clinic, one of my colleagues, Dr. Rekha, encountered Darren* (Name Changed), a 28-year-old seeking a routine check-up. Little did they know, this visit would unfurl a chain of events that would alter Darren's dental journey profoundly.

Darren, unsuspecting of any dental distress, visited Dr Rekha for what he assumed to be a regular check-up. However, Dr Rekha's keen eye detected something amiss in Darren's upper jaw. An incidental finding during the examination revealed a substantial cyst nestled inconspicuously amidst his left upper front teeth, a silent threat unnoticed by Darren.

Further investigation through advanced imaging techniques illuminated the gravity of the situation—the cyst, stemming from prior root canals, had grown to a startling size, concealed from view but silently expanding. The risk was substantial, urging immediate action to prevent potential complications.

Swiftly, the dental team embarked on a meticulous plan. The cyst, despite its significant size, was delicately removed and sent for biopsy—a moment of palpable anxiety that was alleviated when the results returned clear, signalling a crucial victory.

The journey didn't end there. With precision and care, a two-step approach unfolded. Bone grafting filled the void left by the cyst, laying the groundwork for future restoration. Four months later, Dr Rekha skilfully placed two stable dental implants, signalling a promising milestone in Darren's recovery journey.

The procedure didn't merely restore teeth; it rekindled hope and confidence. Darren's healing progress was remarkable, culminating in the placement of temporary crowns, a testament to the success of the intervention. With a zirconia crown on the horizon, Darren's smile was on the path to its former glory.

Moral of the story:

Darren's story vividly illustrates the profound impact of routine dental check-ups. What appeared to be a regular visit unravelled a hidden threat, emphasising the vital role of proactive dental care. The narrative underlines the significance of timely intervention, demonstrating how a simple check-up not only preserved Darren's smile but potentially safeguarded his overall well-being. It illuminates the importance of early detection, proactive treatment, and the invaluable role of dental visits in preserving both smiles and lives.

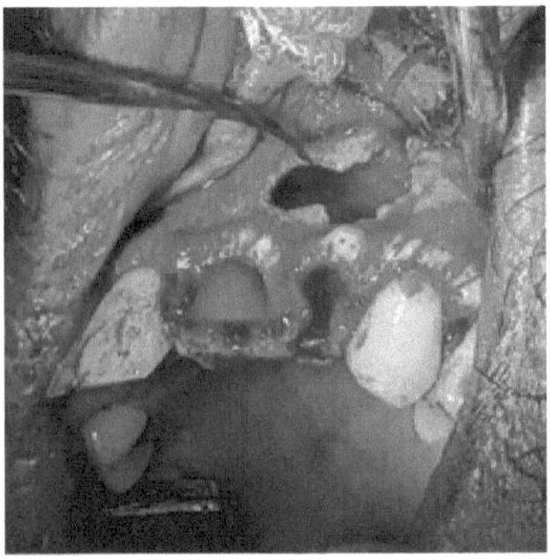

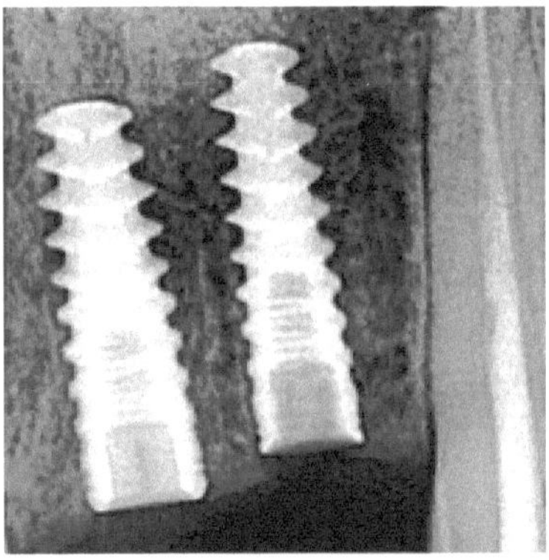

CHAPTER - 44

LOST MOBILE PHONE AND FAILED IMPLANTS

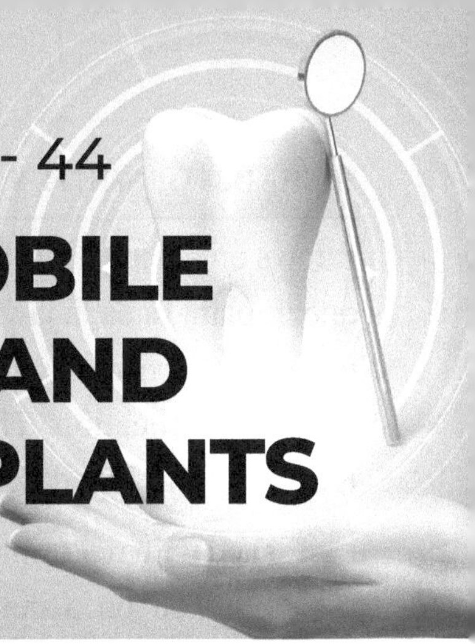

In the intricate tapestry of dental narratives, the tale of Mr Shankar, a 51-year-old from the UK, unfolds as a saga of unexpected challenges, resilience, and redemption. The journey began in 2018 when Mr Shankar opted for the transformative Four Implant procedure. Little did we know that this chapter would take a surprising turn, testing the bonds of communication and the resilience of dental reconstruction.

As is customary in our practice, we extend invitations for annual reviews to ensure the continued well-being of our patients. However, Mr Shankar vanished without a trace after his initial treatment. For years, our attempts to reach him were met with silence. His sudden reappearance in 2023 brought with it an unexpected story - his mobile phone and wallet were stolen on the way to the airport in 2018, rendering him disconnected from our clinic.

Mr. Shankar revealed that during this period of disconnection, a crucial issue had emerged. One of the screws on his implants had loosened, leading to the failure of one implant in each jaw. Remarkably, Mr Shankar continued to use the prosthesis, seemingly oblivious to the evolving dental complication. The consequences were evident – the loosening had failed one more implant in each jaw.

Tasked with restoring Mr. Shankar's smile and oral health, we embarked on a new phase of treatment. Transitioning from All on Four to All on Six, we introduced additional implants and opted for a Zirconia prosthesis. The process aimed not only at redemption but also at reinforcing the importance of regular dental reviews.

This time, Mr Shankar has pledged to remain in touch, vowing to return for annual reviews and staying connected to his dental care.

Moral of the Story

Mr Shankar's story underscores the fragility of communication and the impact of unforeseen circumstances on patient follow-up. The narrative prompts reflection on the significance of maintaining open channels of communication in the ever-evolving landscape of patient care.

The patient's resilience in carrying on despite a loosened implant screw serves as a cautionary tale about the importance of proactive dental care and the consequences of neglect. The transition from All on Four to All on Six becomes a symbol of redemption, emphasising the possibility of corrective measures even after setbacks.

And keep your mobile phones and wallet safe always!!

Before

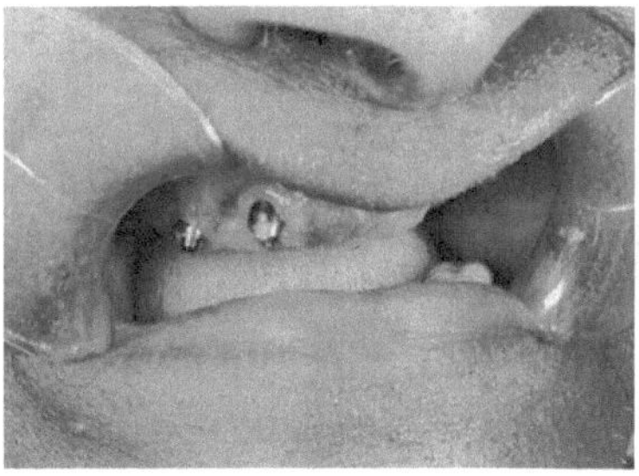

After

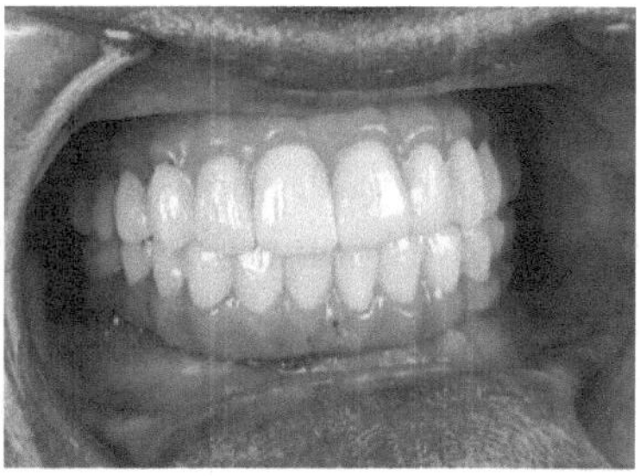

CHAPTER - 45

A PROMISE KEPT - SANJAY'S DENTAL TRIUMPH

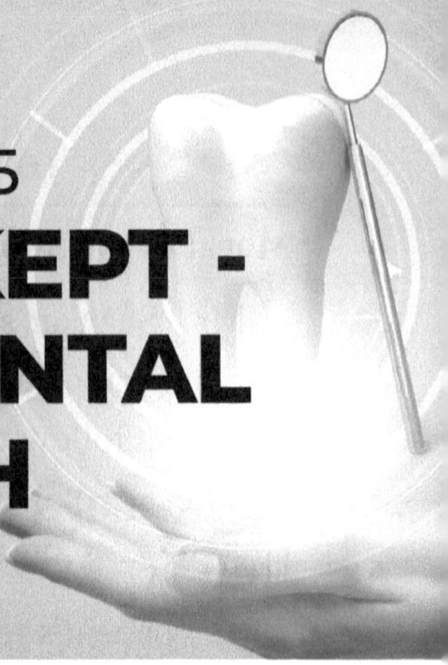

In the unfolding chapters of my dental practice, this poignant story centres around a young soul named Sanjay*(Name Changed). At 23, Sanjay arrived at my clinic in 2022, seeking a solution for his missing upper front teeth. The recommendation was a single implant and crown for immediate restoration, a prospect that excited Sanjay immensely. His eagerness to commence the treatment was evident as he proposed paying 20% as an advance.

However, after this initial burst of enthusiasm, Sanjay seemingly vanished from our radar for six months. The attempts made by my team to reach him were met with silence. It was only upon his return that we learned the reason for his sudden disappearance. Sanjay had been diligently working and saving, ensuring that he had the finances required before proceeding with the surgery.

His determination and sincerity deeply moved my team, realising that Sanjay had gone to great lengths to fulfil his commitment. Had he communicated his financial situation earlier, we would have gladly worked out a flexible payment plan to expedite his treatment. Sanjay's honesty and hard work became the catalyst for us to reassess and accommodate his financial needs.

We decided to split his payments, ensuring that he received the best crowns and paid at his convenience. Money ceased to be a barrier between Sanjay's aspirations for a radiant smile and the quality dental care he deserved.

Moral of the Story:

Sanjay's narrative emphasises the importance of clear communication and understanding between patients and dental care providers. It serves as a reminder that financial constraints should never hinder access to quality dental care, especially for the younger generation.

The moral of the story is twofold. Firstly, young minds with dental aspirations should feel empowered to communicate openly about their financial situations. Dental professionals, on the other hand, should foster an environment that encourages such communication, allowing for tailored solutions that prioritise patient care.

Secondly, the story underscores the need for flexibility in payment plans. By adapting to Sanjay's financial circumstances, we not only fulfilled his dental aspirations but also strengthened the bond of trust between patient and practitioner. Ultimately, the chapter showcases the transformative power of understanding, compassion, and a shared commitment to achieving a bright and confident smile.

CHAPTER - 46

A DECADE UNVEILED - A PERIODONTIST'S FATHER'S DENTAL JOURNEY

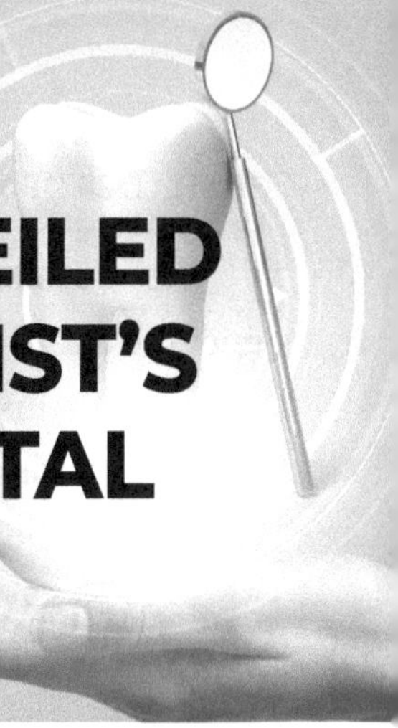

Over a decade, the tale of Saravanan* (Name Changed) unfolds, revealing a remarkable journey in pursuit of renewed smiles. Back in 2012, at the threshold of his senior years, Saravanan embarked on a 250-kilometre journey from his native place to Chennai. Under my care, Seven Implants adorned his upper arch, accompanied by a hybrid prosthesis, while the lower received 2 implants supporting a six-unit bridge in the anterior. The procedure, conducted in my previous role at a different hospital, became a shared chapter in his family's history.

A decade later, in 2022, Saravanan sought me out at Apollo Dental OMR, tracing the footsteps of his dental history. As our paths converged again, the resilience of his implants emerged as a testament to enduring quality. Not a hint of bone loss marred their perfection, and the prosthesis, though exhibiting minor wear, stood resilient against the test of time.

The decade between our encounters saw Saravanan undergo a cardiac bypass surgery, a testament to the profound changes in his life. Meanwhile, his daughters flourished, both graduating as doctors. One chose the path of paediatric care, while the other, like me, became a Periodontist.

Presenting with pain in his lower back teeth, Saravanan entrusted me once more with his oral health. Despite his cardiac history, extraction became a necessary step, executed after meticulous consent from his cardiologist. Four additional implants found their place in the lower arch, and the opportunity to elevate his smiles beckoned. We transitioned his upper prosthesis to a resplendent zirconia masterpiece, mirroring the transformation in his lower arch.

With every appointment, Saravanan brings his Periodontist daughter, eager to learn the art of implant dentistry. And I have promised his daughter a job in my implant team once she finishes her course.

Moral of the Story

Saravanan's journey reflects the enduring nature of meticulous dental care and the transformative power of advancements in prosthodontics. The tale underscores the importance of long-term follow-up and the resilience of well-planned implant procedures.

Before

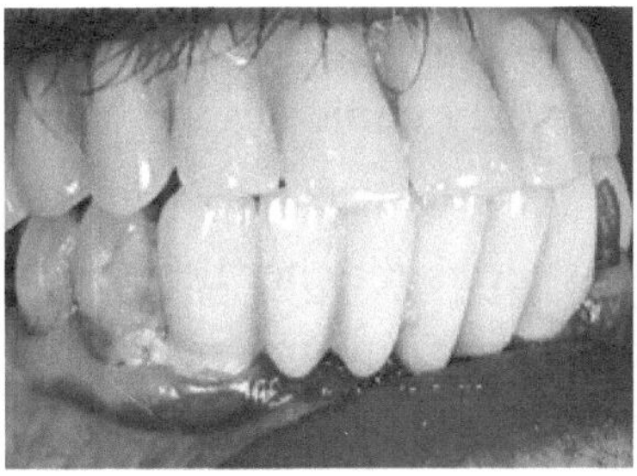

After

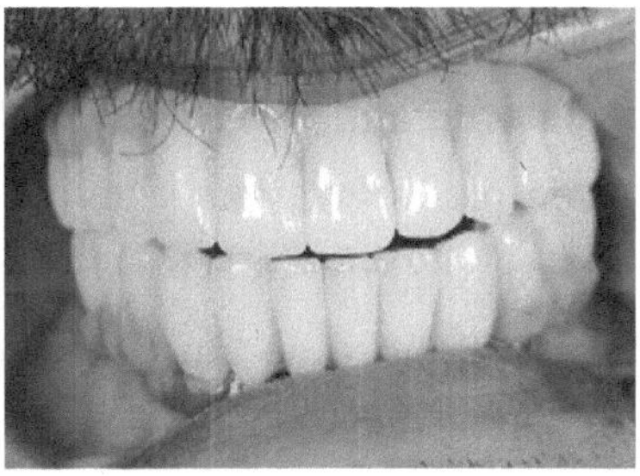

CHAPTER - 47

FAITH BEYOND DISTANCE

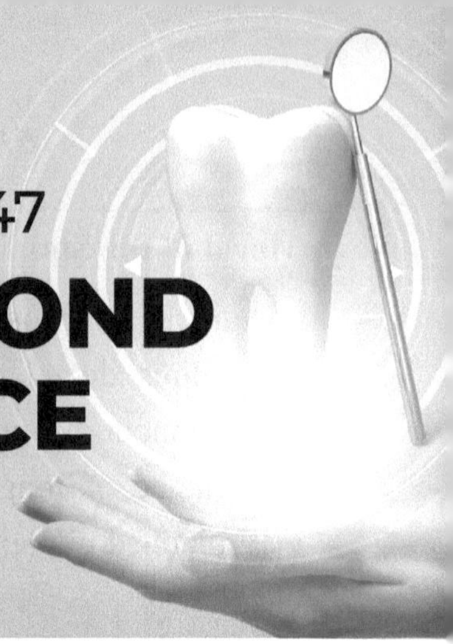

In the vast landscape of dental transformations, the remarkable journey of Meena* (Name Changed), a 66-year-old lady from Trichy*(City Changed), unfolds as a testament to unwavering faith and commitment. Discovered through my YouTube videos, Meena's decision to undergo implant treatment led her to choose my clinic despite being seven hours away and having known dentists closer to her. The most surprising twist in this tale is that her nephew, a Prosthodontist and my mentor during my undergraduate days, was overlooked in favour of me.

From the outset, Meena and her family exhibited extraordinary faith and trust in me. Despite the distance and the availability of family connections in the dental field, Meena chose to fly for hours to every appointment at my clinic. The decision to bypass local dentists and her own nephew showcased a profound trust that transcended geographical boundaries.

Embarking on a comprehensive implant journey, we placed 6 implants in the upper arch and 5 in the lower arch, providing Meena with an immediate prosthesis. Though the initial prosthesis didn't entirely meet her expectations, Meena held steadfast faith in me, understanding that the final outcome would be nothing short of excellent.

For Meena, the climax of her journey was marked by the creation of a Malo Bridge featuring a Titanium bar and Zirconia crowns in the final prosthesis after a meticulous 4-month wait. The joy radiated not just from her but also from her delighted family, and Meena emerged as a patient who not only took her yearly reviews seriously but also cherished the transformed smile she waited for.

Moral of the story:

Meena's story underscores the profound impact of trust and faith in the patient-dentist relationship. The narrative emphasises that quality of care and the rapport established during treatment can transcend geographic proximity and familial connections.

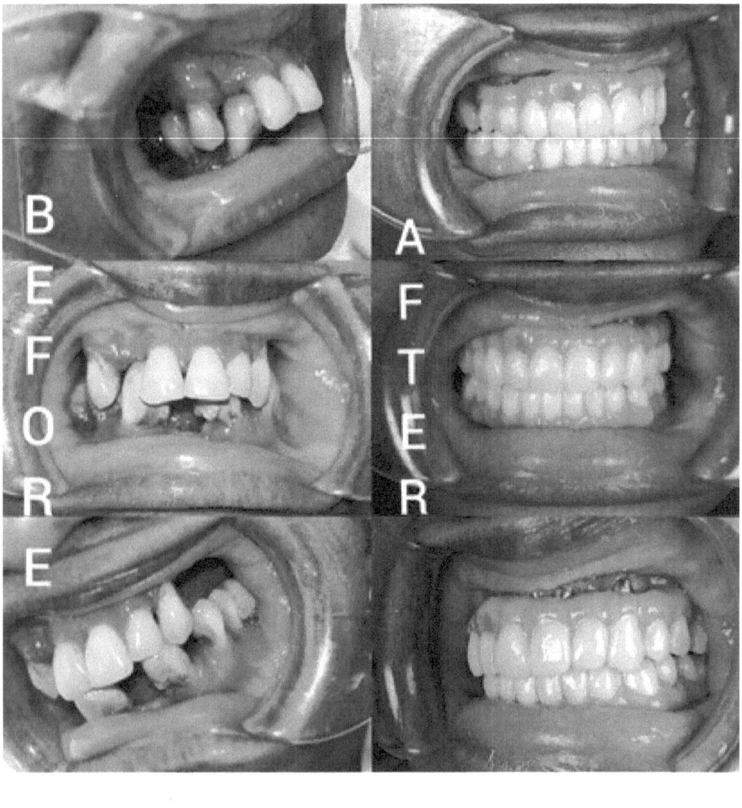

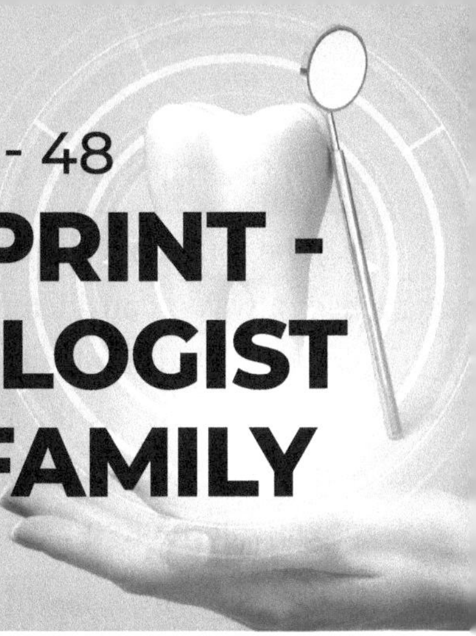

CHAPTER - 48

FATE'S IMPRINT - IMPLANTOLOGIST FOR THE FAMILY

A unique story unfolds, weaving together the lives of a husband and wife in unexpected ways. Back in 2010, the husband sought my expertise for multiple failing bridges, leading to a comprehensive restoration involving sinus lifts and crowns. Over the years, he made frequent visits for reviews, always accompanied by his wife. Surprisingly, though, she never sought a consultation.

Fast forward to 2020, and fate took me to Madurai for a consulting opportunity at a hospital. To my astonishment, one of the cases presented was the wife of this longstanding patient. Despite being in my office countless times, she had never taken a step towards a consultation until her husband chose to pursue dental implants for her.

The husband, visibly embarrassed, explained that he had always considered bridges for his wife and never contemplated implants until then. The unexpected twist of fate placed me as the implantologist for both husband and wife. He expressed his relief and happiness at the fortuitous alignment of circumstances.

For the wife's case, I placed 2 implants in her upper front teeth and provided temporary teeth within 30 minutes. The husband and wife, now both beneficiaries of dental implants, shared a sense of contentment and gratitude.

Moral of the story:

In the realm of dentistry, it reminds us that patients may take their time to decide on comprehensive treatment plans. The husband's journey from bridges to embracing dental implants for his wife underscores the transformative power of informed decision-making. Ultimately, the chapter imparts the moral that, sometimes, fate plays a role in uniting patients and practitioners on unexpected yet fulfilling journeys.

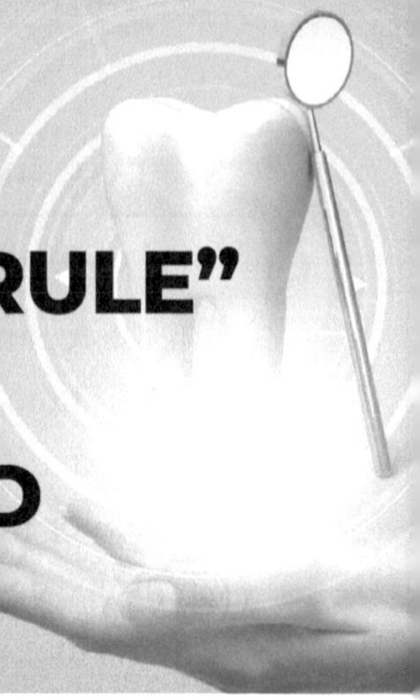

CHAPTER - 49
"THE FIVE YEAR RULE" AND THE 40-YEAR-OLD

In the chronicles of dental transformations, the narrative of Rajan* (Name Changed), a 40-year-old seeking solace from multiple loose teeth, emerges as a testimony to the power of comprehensive oral care. In 2022, he entered our clinic, facing a critical juncture in his oral health — a borderline scenario where the decision hovered between a full mouth implant approach and an intricate gum treatment coupled with multiple implants.

Adhering to a principle known as the "5-year rule," I evaluated each tooth's viability, contemplating whether it could serve its function for the next five years. For Rajan, this assessment revealed that most of his teeth fell short of the 5-year rule, necessitating their removal for a more sustainable and functionally enhanced solution. The recommended course of action was all-encompassing — full mouth implants.

With resilience and readiness, Rajan embraced the proposed treatment plan, envisioning not just restored oral health but a smile that reflected his aspirations. His specific desire for high-quality Zirconia teeth prompted the selection of the All On Four Implants approach. After an 8-week anticipation period, the journey culminated in the crafting of a Malo Bridge adorned with Zirconia teeth.

What made this odyssey truly special was the unwavering support of Rajan's father-in-law, a pillar of encouragement throughout the surgery and the entire treatment process. The camaraderie extended beyond clinical walls, fostering a bond that transcended patient-practitioner dynamics.

The completion of Rajan's treatment marked not just the revival of a healthy and functional smile but the birth of a lasting friendship. Rajan, now a brand ambassador, reflects the transformative impact of full mouth implants not only on oral health but also on one's overall well-being.

Moral of the story:

Rajan's story illuminates the significance of timely and comprehensive dental care, demonstrating how adherence to principled decision-making can lead to transformative outcomes. The 5-year rule serves as a guiding principle, ensuring that patients like Rajan receive solutions that stand the test of time.

Be like Rajan!

CHAPTER - 50

THE SOUTH AFRICAN'S SAFARI TO INDIA FOR A CONFIDENT SMILE

In the bustling world of Marketing, where first impressions are pivotal, Mr. Morgan, a seasoned professional in a multinational company in Durban, South Africa, found himself at a crossroads. A childhood marked by dental challenges had left him with only two front teeth in the upper jaw, casting a shadow over his confidence during client meetings and sales endeavours. The constant extraction of teeth had taken a toll, and Morgan yearned for a solution that would restore not just his teeth but also his self-assurance.

The turning point came during the era of Covid-19, a period Morgan considered a blessing in disguise. The ubiquitous masks offered him a temporary shield, allowing him to venture out without revealing his dental concerns. Yet, deep down, he knew that a more permanent solution was necessary. After contemplating for over a year, Morgan made the courageous decision to seek dental treatment in India, with me as his chosen Implantologist.

Morgan, accompanied by his supportive wife, embarked on a transformative journey to my clinic. The treatment plan involved Six Implants in the upper arch, complemented by an immediate Hybrid prosthesis, and multiple implants in the lower arch with Zirconia crowns. To enhance precision and minimise invasiveness, we opted for keyhole surgery, a technique that significantly reduces bleeding and eliminates the need for sutures.

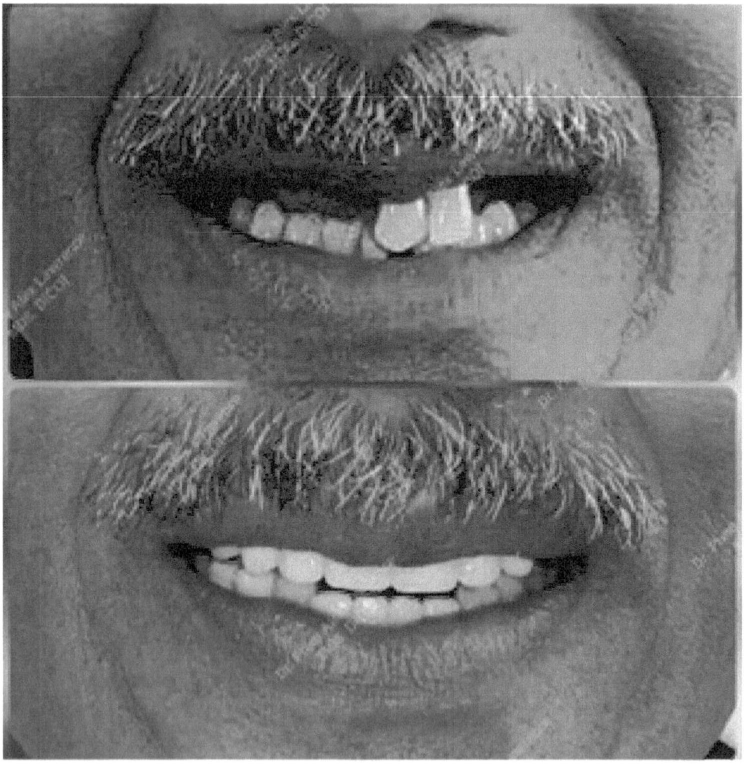

Between appointments, Morgan and his wife explored the rich cultural tapestry of India, visiting the Temple Town Mahabalipuram and the serene Aurobindo Ashram in Pondicherry. They indulged in some shopping in T Nagar, making the most of their time in India.

The climax of Morgan's journey unfolded on the day of crown delivery. Mrs. Morgan, overwhelmed with emotion, shared a tight hug and a kiss, exclaiming that the "Old Morgan" was back. A video call to their children captured the moment, and the joy reflected on their faces was evident. Morgan returned to South Africa not just with a revitalised smile but with renewed confidence, ready to engage with clients and colleagues without the weight of dental concerns.

Moral of the story:

Morgan's story encapsulates the profound impact of dental transformations on one's self-esteem and professional confidence. It underscores the significance of making decisions that not only address immediate concerns but also pave the way for long-term well-being.

Morgan's odyssey serves as an inspiration, illustrating that a comprehensive dental solution can be the key to reclaiming not just one's smile but also the assurance to face the world with renewed vigour and confidence.

To watch a video of the full story of Mr Morgan

Made in United States
Troutdale, OR
11/03/2026

56845270R00106